FROM BLACK CODES TO RECODIFICATION:

Removing the Veil from Regulatory Writing

Miriam F. Williams
Texas State University

Baywood's Technical Communications Series
Series Editor: CHARLES H. SIDES

Baywood Publishing Company, Inc.
AMITYVILLE, NEW YORK

Copyright © 2010 by Baywood Publishing Company, Inc., Amityville, New York

All rights reserved. No part of this book may be reproduced or utilized in any form or by any means, electronic or mechanical, including photo-copying, recording, or by any information storage or retrieval system, without permission in writing from the publisher. Printed in the United States of America on acid-free recycled paper.

Baywood Publishing Company, Inc.
26 Austin Avenue
P.O. Box 337
Amityville, NY 11701
(800) 638-7819
E-mail: baywood@baywood.com
Web site: baywood.com

Library of Congress Catalog Number: 2009029839
ISBN: 978–0–89503–376–5 (cloth)

Library of Congress Cataloging-in-Publication Data

Williams, Miriam F.
   From Black codes to recodification : removing the veil from regulatory writing / Miriam Williams.
       p. cm. -- (Baywood's technical communications series)
   Includes bibliographical references and index.
   ISBN 978–0–89503–376–5 (cloth : alk. paper)
   1. Technical writing. 2. Communication of technical information. 3. African Americans--Texas--History. I. Title.
   T11.W52 2009
   323.1196'0730764--dc22

                                                        2009029839

Table of Contents

ACKNOWLEDGMENTS v

CHAPTER I. Introduction: Race, Regulations, and Trust 1

    Traditional Styles of Regulatory Writing 3
    Contemporary Arguments for Plain English Regulations 6
    Organization of Book 8

**CHAPTER II. Case Study I—Texas Black Codes of 1866:
Identifying Discourse Markers of Trust** 15

    Identifying Discourse Markers of Trust 17
    Discourse Analysis of Texas Black Codes 22
    Findings of Discourse Analysis 24

**CHAPTER III. Texas Laws and Tacit Laws: Redefining Black
Labor from "The Nadir" to Civil Rights** 35

    Redefining Apprenticeship and Contract Labor 42
    Rationale for Contemporary Studies 46

**CHAPTER IV. Case Study II—Texas Agencies: The Challenge
of Evoking Trust** 49

    Contextual Inquiry Meeting at State Agency 50
    Artifacts Collected during Contextual Inquiry Study 52
    Process Meeting with Group of Policy Writers 52
    Analysis of Regulatory Writing Tasks 53

**CHAPTER V. Case Study III—Contemporary Black Business
Owners: Legalese, Plain English, or Both?** 67

    The Focus Group in Context 72

CHAPTER VI. An Invention Heuristic for Regulatory Writing 79

    Implications of Contextual Inquiry and Focus Group Studies 80
    What Information Do New Policy Writers Need to Know? 82
    What Style Meets the Needs of the Government Agency and
        the Public? 83
    A Rulemaking Heuristic to Evoke Trust in Distrustful Audiences 86
    Considerations for the Future of Regulatory Writing 89

APPENDICES
    Appendix I: Texas Black Codes in Legalese and Plain English 93
    Appendix II: Rhetorical Analysis of Texas Black Codes in
        Legalese and Plain English 111
    Appendix III: Contextual Inquiry Transcript 129
    Appendix IV: The Focus Group Meeting 139

REFERENCES 149
INDEX 157

Acknowledgments

I thank my former professors in Texas Tech University's Technical Communication and Rhetoric Program for their guidance, feedback and encouragement; my colleagues in Texas State University's Department of English for their continued support; and my former colleagues at the State of Texas for introducing me to regulatory writing. Most important, I would like to thank my family and friends for their prayers and encouragement. Specifically, I thank Thereisa Coleman and Marcia Williams for reading and editing several drafts of this manuscript. I would also like to thank Charles Sides and the Baywood editing and production staff for their patience and commitment to this project.

CHAPTER I

Introduction: Race, Regulations, and Trust

In *The Souls of Black Folk* (2003), W. E. B. DuBois wields two of the most powerful metaphors of the Gilded Age, the "veil" and the "color line." In this work, DuBois, a sociologist, provides sociological and historical accounts of African American life after Reconstruction. Recurring throughout DuBois' essays in *The Souls of Black Folk,* whether political, sociological, or biographical, are his references to the impact of the "veil" and "color line" on African American life, and how "black folk" across socioeconomic and regional lines have responded to the realities of living in a society with a legally protected color line. Emory Elliot further explores these metaphors in his article, "The Veil, the Mask, and the Invisible Empire: Representations of Race in the Gilded Age" (1989) and provides evidence of how language was used to veil discriminatory practices against African Americans in the dissemination of one of America's more treasured art forms, literature (pp. 11–17). Elliot rests on Houston Baker's description of DuBois' veil—"a barrier of American racial segregation that keeps Afro-Americans always behind a color line—disoriented prey to divided aims, dire economic circumstances, haphazard educational opportunities and frustrated intellectual ambitions"—to support his argument (cited in Elliot, 1989, p. 16). Much of Elliot's article examines how race was portrayed in the works of Herman Melville and white authors, including Mark Twain, who examined race relations in a more realistic context than most white authors (pp. 12–14). Elliot's main argument is that white authors, including Herman Melville, may have veiled characters such as Billy Budd and Claggart in allegory to steer clear of the political ramifications of painting a realistic image of racism in America (p. 13). While Cornell West (2004) regards Melville's works as "an unprecedented and unmatched meditation on the imperialist and racist impediments to democracy in American life," (p. 87), Emory Elliot asks, "Is it possible that in the 1880's and 90's even Melville had to insinuate the racial implications of his work in such subtle ways that they are nearly invisible?" (1989, p. 13).

Melville's need to veil antislavery rhetoric in allegory could be linked to his familial relationship with one of its strongest proponents; West explains that Melville's father-in-law was "the judge who sustained the Fugitive Slave Act that was a catalyst for the Civil War" (2004, p. 48). According to Elliot, the color line helped shape the figurative language we find in some of our most highly regarded literary works (1989, p. 15). Certainly, if we examine the rhetorical situations surrounding the invention of these works, we'll find that African Americans were not considered as members of the audience who read these works, and thus it was easy to distort their images and reality. During this same period, in government laws and regulations, the Western style of writing, which has rhetorical roots dating as far back as ancient Greek and Roman societies, created the perfect construct for a similar veil that masked discriminatory laws and ordinances in detached, complex, and jargon-filled language that we now call "legalese." I am not arguing that legalese was used to evade any powerful voices of African Americans, many of whom could not read or obtain legal texts, but I am arguing that the style of writing used in historical regulations directed at African American audiences served the same purpose as Melville's allegory. While Melville's allegory served as a veil to his attacks on racism in America, regulatory writing veiled consistent attacks on the civil rights of African Americans. During this period in American history, language was used to veil mentions of race and racial discrimination in both literature and law. While Emory Elliot explains that there was an "absence of race from American text [literature] in the period" (1989, p. 15), Barry Crouch adds that Texas Black Codes of 1866 "appeared to ignore race" (1999, p. 264). Still, we know that racially discriminatory laws and regulations directed at African Americans were promulgated from Antebellum to Jim Crow. David Bernstein (2001) noted the continuation of this writing style throughout the southern states and argued, "facially neutral occupational regulations passed between the 1870s and the 1930s harmed African Americans. Sometimes racism motivated the laws, either directly (as when the sponsors of the legislation were themselves racists) or indirectly (when legislative sponsors responded to racism among their constituents)" (p. 5) (Crouch, 1999, p. 264). These authors suggest that writers of Texas Black Codes and labor regulation writers after Reconstruction used veiled language to intentionally mask discrimination against African Americans in regulations. Thus, the "racially neutral" style of labor regulations that intentionally hid the intended black audience was an official veil that perpetuated African American "disorientation, dire economic circumstances, and frustration" that defines DuBois' color line (cited in Elliot, 1989, p. 16). Now, decades after the dismantling of most legalized discrimination against African Americans, ambiguous regulations persist and in this book, I posit that many historically marginalized groups, including African Americans, are resistant to the traditional style of regulatory writing, not because they cannot read regulations or hire attorneys to interpret these texts, but because written laws represent a veil that for so many years acted as a rhetorical accomplice to America's color line. Although regulatory writing has a long history dating back centuries before America and its laws, regulations like the Texas Black Codes and post-Reconstruction labor laws have so tainted the African American audience's perception of legal discourse, that regulations are perceived, not simply as the traditional style for this genre, but as a style that evokes distrust.

TRADITIONAL STYLES OF REGULATORY WRITING

Concerns for regulatory writing invention and style did not begin with Barry Crouch or assessments of the intent of Texas Black Codes, which were obviously in conflict with the language used to convey the law, but with classical rhetoricians who also debated these issues with particular emphasis on the roles of clarity and ambiguity in regulatory writing. Before we can look for a style of regulatory writing that evokes trust, we must examine the goals of regulatory writers. In *Rulemaking: How Government Agencies Write Law and Make Policy,* Cornelius M. Kerwin argues, "writers have three distinct goals for writing regulations, to implement, interpret and prescribe" (1994, p. 5). Kerwin states that regulation*s* "interpret when law and policy are well established but confront unanticipated but changing circumstances," "prescribe when Congress establishes the goals of law or policy in statutes but provides few details as to how they are to be put into operation," and "implement when law or policy has been fully developed in Congress, an executive order of the president, or judicial decision" (pp. 5–6). There are inconsistencies as well as intersections between Kerwin's goals for regulatory writers and the styles of writing advocated by proponents of the user-centered Plain English style and the traditional "legalese" style.

Since both Technical Communication and Public Policy research depend on classical rhetoricians for insight into the invention of democracies and the laws that govern them, it is important to begin our examination into regulatory writing by discussing their early contributions to this genre. The classical rhetoricians provide us with no consensus regarding the most appropriate style for writing laws in ancient Greece and Rome. In *The Laws,* Plato uses a dialogue between Cleinias and the Athenian to argue for specificity in written laws and suggests that ambiguous words must be defined in laws. In this dialogue the Athenian states, "But you ought not to use the term 'moderate' in the way you did just now; you must say what 'moderate' means and how big or small it may be. If you don't you must realize that a remark such as you made still has some way to go before it can be law" (1970, p. 181). In *The Orator,* Cicero argues that conflicts arise "out of the construction of a document, wherein there is some ambiguity or contradiction, or something is so expressed that the written word is in variance with the intention" (1988, p. 99). Cicero reiterates this point in *The Laws* while simultaneously contradicting Plato's argument about specificity that leads to confusion. In Cicero's *The Laws,* he criticizes legal experts by stating, "But legal experts, whether to cause confusion and so give the appearance of having a wider and deeper knowledge than they do, or (more probably) through their incompetence at putting the subject across (for an art is not just a matter of knowing something; it is also a matter of communication) often endlessly subdivide a thing which is based on a single idea" (1998, p. 141). Here, we find both Plato and Cicero arguing against ambiguity; Plato argues for clarity through meticulous definitions or subdivisions as we find in legalese, while Cicero argues for further clarity through the avoidance of Plato's definitions and subdivisions, which manifest in complex clauses and lengthy sentences. Cicero's suggestion is also supported by Plain Language advocates. In contrast to both Plato and Cicero's views, in *On Rhetoric,* Aristotle asserts that "If, then, the action is undefinable when a law must be framed, it is necessary to speak in general terms, so that if someone wearing a ring raises his hand or strikes, by the written law is violating the law and does wrong, when in truth he has [perhaps] not done any harms, and this [after judgment] is fair" (1991, p. 105). In his usual manner, Aristotle considers occasions where the opposite may also be appropriate when he states "[it] is highly appropriate for well-enacted laws to define everything as exactly as possible and for as little as possible to be left to the judges" (p. 31). In the first quote, Aristotle argues for a style of legal writing that leaves room for ambiguity and interpretation so that regulations are still enforceable when the unforeseen crime or illegality occurs, but in his second quote he claims that there are situations when regulations should be as specific as possible. These statements, like Aristotle's common places, are evidence of his advocacy for considering the "available means of persuasion in each case" (p. 35).

Other recommendations from classical Greek rhetoricians that do not speak directly to the writing of laws or regulations, but do pertain to the appropriateness of certain styles of writing given specific situations are found in Demetrius' *On Style.* George Kennedy describes Demetrius' work as the "earliest surviving monographic treatment of style in which Demetrius discusses the plain, grand, elegant, and forceful" styles of rhetoric (1994, p. 89). In yet another discussion of these types of style, the author of *Rhetorica ad Herennium Book IV,* whom Kennedy states is possibly Cornificius or Cicero but is often credited as "Anonymous," discusses three kinds of style: the grand, the middle, and the simple. In this text, the author states that "the grand style consists of smooth and ornate arrangement of impressive words" appropriate for appeals to pity and amplification, "the middle consist of words of lower, yet not of the lowest and most colloquial class of words" and "the simple type is brought down even to the most current idiom of standard speech" (Bizzell & Herzberg, 2001, p. 248; Kennedy, 1994, p. 121). More importantly for this study, the classical rhetorician argues "clarity renders language plain and intelligible. It is achieved by two means, the use of current terms and of proper terms. Current terms are such as are habitually used in everyday speech. Proper terms are, or can be, the designations specifically characteristic of the subject of discourse" (Bizzell & Herzberg, 2001, p. 248). In this statement, the author does not explicitly equate clarity with the simple style, but suggests that clarity and the simple style do share one feature, "current terms," whereas "proper terms" are not necessarily a part of the simple or plain style.

These classical rhetoricians give us four stylistic choices for regulatory writing: (1) Plato suggests that regulatory writers be very detailed in an effort to avoid ambiguity; (2) Cicero tells regulatory writers to be clear and brief to avoid ambiguity; (3) Aristotle suggests that regulatory writers be general, even ambiguous, to allot for unexpected circumstances, but also states that there are situations where specificity is appropriate, yet he stops short of arguing for clarity; and (4) the author of *Rhetorica ad Herennium* defines clarity as more than plain language, but correct and specific language. The intersection of these recommendations, three of which pertain specifically to written laws, is clarity—while some suggest means of achieving it, others attempt to define it or avoid it entirely. While Plato and Cicero take a more positivist approach, Aristotle seems to rest on a postmodern perspective of written laws in that he does not argue for clarity (Walzer & Gross, 1994, p. 421). In "Positivists, Postmodernists, Aristotelians, and the Challenger Disaster," Arthur E. Walzer and Alan Gross argue that technical communicators who analyzed the Challenger space shuttle disaster relied on three forms of analysis: a positivist approach, which suggests that the disaster occurred because information was not clear or transparent; a postmodern approach, which suggests that in the debates leading up to the disaster "no 'facts' speak for themselves; meaning comes only with interpretation; language can never be a transparent medium of reality," and an Aristotelian approach that considers that there could be more than one possible argument or rationale for the disaster (p. 422). Walzer and Gross propose that the most appropriate type of analysis for understanding the disaster would be a rhetorical analysis or an Aristotelian analysis that examines two possibilities, and they quote Aristotle in stating that "the purpose of rhetorical deliberation is to discover the best available means of persuasion" (p. 426). Certainly, Aristotle's suggestion for regulatory writing to leave room for other possibilities and also to be as specific as possible does not contradict Walzer and Gross' interpretation of an Aristotelian perspective.

Given the goals of regulations, which Kerwin states are to implement, interpret and prescribe (1994, p. 5), we can surmise that regulatory writing calls for different styles and perspectives, depending on the purpose of a particular regulation. The first goal in regulatory writing is to "interpret when law and policy are well established but confront unanticipated but changing circumstances" (p. 5). To meet the demands of this goal, we can rely on one of Aristotle's suggestions, which is to apply general and vague language to allot room for the unexpected violations. The second goal of regulatory writing is to "prescribe when Congress establishes the goals of law or policy in statutes but provides few details as to how they are to be put into operation" (p. 5). In meeting this goal, the regulation writer is charged with adding more specific language or definitions as proposed by Plato and also Aristotle (in his second recommendation), employing a positivist perspective. Finally, the third goal of regulatory writing is to "implement, when law or policy has been fully developed in Congress, an executive order of the president, or judicial decision" (p. 5). In such cases, where the regulatory actions are "fully" explained by some other authorizing body, whether it be Congress or the executive or judicial branches, agencies would be justified in simply revising or clarifying these inherited mandates into regulations and applying the definition of clarification provided by the author of *Rhetorica ad Herennium:* "the use of current terms and of proper terms" to aid in the delicate tasks of policy implementation (Bizzell & Herzberg, 2001, p. 248). In this case, regulatory writers must resort to a postmodern perspective in that "proper terms" are subjective. Clearly, these suggestions are an amalgam of the recommendations made by proponents of the Plain English style and the legalese style. The classical rhetoricians argue that, depending on the situation or goal of the writer, there is a time and place for various styles of regulatory writing.

Although the classical rhetoricians were concerned with regulatory language, intent, and *kairos* and it is obvious that their recommendations influenced the Western tradition of regulatory writing, the consideration of written laws that evoke trust or distrust in historically marginalized groups is a 20th-century phenomenon.

CONTEMPORARY ARGUMENTS FOR PLAIN ENGLISH REGULATIONS

In 1998, Vice President Gore announced the Plain Language in Government Writing Executive Memorandum, issued by then-President Bill Clinton and later attended a Plain English awards ceremony where Gore explained, "Plain language helps create understanding, and understanding helps create trust. And trust—especially trust in the promise of self-government—is essential to solving the common problems we face" (Gore, 1998, p. 1). As a result of the Plain Language in Government Writing Executive Memorandum, the Plain English Movement officially resurfaced in the United States government at the federal and states levels (Plainlanguage.gov, 2005). Now, although proponents of Plain English are targeting federal agencies, they are finding support among many state legislators as well. In some states, elected officials have promulgated laws that mandate the rewrite of thousands of regulations, forms, letters, and Web site materials in Plain English. Federal and state agency officials are looking to scholars to define Plain English and to teach public-policy writers how to translate complex legal documents from legalese to Plain English.

In 1999, during the 76th Texas legislative session, the state legislature passed Senate Bill 178, which required a review of all agency regulations to determine if the rationale for promulgating them still existed; this bill served as an impetus for several state agencies to begin not only a review of agency regulations but a rewrite of regulations from legalese to Plain English to increase readability and to decrease ongoing criticism from the public and state legislators. One agency division, the Texas Department of Family and Protective Services' (formerly known as Texas Department of Protective and Regulatory Service) Child Care Licensing Division, initiated a massive rewrite of its agency rules that continues today and serves as a model for other agency rule rewrites.

Two years later, during the 77th Texas Legislative Session, a State of Texas legislator drafted a bill proposing that readability tests be used to evaluate state regulations and publications. This bill, House Bill 3411, included a proposed readability formula that if passed would require state agencies to rewrite all regulations that did not meet the readability standards in the proposed bill. Ironically, the proposed bill, which was critical of state agencies' use of complex style, included less-than-citizen-friendly language in its clause—the process of testing and rewriting the regulations was called "recodification" and the bill was written in classic legalese. The recodification bill died in committee within weeks of its proposal, but the negative perceptions about regulatory writing that inspired the bill persist.

In an effort to dispel these negative perceptions, some Texas agencies currently making the transition from legalese to Plain English began their rewrites without conducting quantitative or qualitative research regarding the effectiveness of Plain English regulations and without evaluating which style of writing is actually preferred by their audiences. Still, in most state agencies in Texas and nationwide, there is consensus; Plain English is better, and few public-policy writers or legislators question this unempirical assessment. In this book, I present case studies that (1) present a historical argument for why African Americans are distrustful of regulatory writing, (2) evaluate contemporary regulatory writers' perceptions of their writing styles and audiences, and (3) test contemporary African American perceptions of two styles of regulatory writing. My rationale for selecting African American laborers and business owners as my sample group is not based on the percentage of businesses owned by this group but on this group's history of advocacy against discriminatory laws. I am suggesting that if government agencies can make rhetorical choices to evoke trust in regulations among African Americans, a group that has a history of political disenfranchisement by government entities and regulations, similar rhetorical and user-centered strategies could be used to evoke trust to an even wider, more accommodating audience.

To this end, this book examines Texas regulations dating as far back as the Texas Black Codes of 1866 (some of the most deceptive regulations in Texas history) to contemporary Texas Child Care Licensing regulations, which quite possibly symbolize some of the most audience-friendly contemporary regulations Texas has to offer. This book also examines the contemporary African American audience, an audience that scholars from political science, categorize as an audience that is distrustful of the government (National Public Radio, 2000, p. 1). My rationale for looking at two extremes of regulatory discourse spanning years of Texas history is to highlight regulatory invention and style in a relatively closed system from 1866 to post-Reconstruction labor regulations, where public comment and input from the true public was not obvious for some, and our current means of inventing regulations in a somewhat open system, where public comments and public opinion about the content and styles of regulations is more obvious. Just as clinical trials test patient responses to new medications during various stages of an injury or illness, the case studies presented in this book test the effects of contemporary Plain English translation on the various stages of regulatory writing, with the Texas Black Codes representing the most severe case of injury and the Child Care Licensing regulations representing a much healthier system. Although the discourse examined in this study is different in style and invention, the user groups examined are African American contracting parties whose work or labor is regulated by government entities. In this book, a discourse analysis of historical regulations and contextual inquiry into contemporary public-policy writing will show how regulation invention has evolved and how changes in these processes impacts the perceptions of a contemporary African American audience—an audience with an oral tradition for whom regulations were an introduction to technical documents and an audience obviously and negatively impacted by historical regulations.

ORGANIZATION OF BOOK

In this chapter, I've attempted to explain the significance of this problem in its historical context. In discussing the limits of historical research, Paul Dombrowski, in Survey of Ethics in Communication and Rhetoric posits, "We should understand that historical views are relevant to us only in broad terms," but argues that we err if we rely too heavily on history to explain contemporary circumstances (2000, p. 14). The federal and state government's contemporary response to this historical problem of ambiguous and deceptive regulations is the promulgation of plain language regulations. Unfortunately little, if any, research has been conducted that shows a causal relationship between Plain English regulations and trust in those groups least trustful of the government, historically marginalized groups. Thus, answers to the questions posed in this book rely heavily on data collected about the invention of contemporary regulations and the perceptions of African American business owners in the present day. The main questions that I am addressing are, Do contemporary Plain English regulations increase trust in African American audiences? Is

Plain English more effective than legalese, which was used to hide discriminatory intent in historical regulations? These questions explore the intercultural conflicts contemporary regulatory writers face in their dual roles as technical communicator/advocate and technical communicator/regulator. The answers to these questions will help to identify what knowledge is privileged in regulation invention and writing processes currently employed by regulatory writers that may include or exclude historically marginalized voices. To find responses to these questions, I present the following chapters:

In Chapter II, I introduce you to some of the most ambiguous and discriminatory regulations in Texas history. Specifically, I present a case study of postbellum Texas Black Codes, regulations written in the late 1800s that allowed white landowners to contract the labor of recently freed blacks and their children under terms that eerily resembled slavery. I conducted this case study to determine if the language, tone, and style used in these regulations would evoke trust in a rational audience. The results of this case study reveal that there are certain rhetorical and stylistic choices evident in the legalese style of these regulations that make some of Texas' most deceptive regulations even more deceptive. A detailed historical and discourse analysis of the Texas Black Codes found in Appendices I and II of this book reveal that historical regulations, even if translated into the Plain English style, can be deceptive and evoke distrust if critical data informed by the historical, social, political, or economic contexts in which regulations are invented are intentionally or unintentionally left out of the regulation.

In Chapter III, I examine early attempts by Texans to disseminate plain language regulations to laypersons via another form of technical communication: manuals. These plain language manuals were addressed to Texas farmers, an audience that included African American sharecroppers. In comparing Texas laws from 1906 and 1921 with "made plain" versions of the same laws, I discovered that the plain language manuals actually included some information that had been repealed years earlier by the Texas Legislature. In addition to plain language laws, I discuss how tacit laws were also used as an extension of codified laws to discriminate against black laborers as they attempted to acquire trades and business ownership.

In Chapter IV, I move my focus from the text of regulations to writers of regulations. I recount my interviews and observations of contemporary State of Texas regulatory writers and unveil the rhetorical strategies that they use to persuade multicultural and distrustful audiences. (A transcript of these interviews are found in Appendix III). This case study reveals that contemporary regulatory writers are conditioned to consider more than their "addressed" audience; there is also a voiceless "invoked" audience, who will never read the regulation, yet whose voices should certainly be considered (Ede & Lunsford, 1997, pp. 78–83). Contemporary regulatory writers consider and address both those protected by the regulations and those required to read and comply with the regulations. This portion of the study also revealed areas where regulatory writers need guidance and instruction from technical communicators to write effective regulations for multicultural audiences.

In Chapter V, I examine the audience for contemporary regulations and describe the findings of a focus group meeting that I held with African American business owners in Austin, Texas and their responses to the two styles of regulations: Plain English and legalese. This portion of the research does reveal that African American business owners are still distrustful of the government, but the Plain English style of writing is effective in evoking trust in this audience. While some of their responses were insightful and useful for technical communicators interested in evoking trust in historically distrustful audiences, some responses revealed deep social wounds that government agencies cannot resolve through written discourse and communication. A transcript of the entire focus group meeting is found in Appendix IV.

In Chapter VI, I conclude by compiling the findings of the case studies, which examine the regulatory texts, policy writers, and audience, into an invention heuristic that can be used by regulatory writers when addressing audiences who are distrustful. More importantly, this apparatus may be used to develop a new style of regulatory writing that responds to the needs of the regulatory agency and the audience and forces the regulatory writer to consider culture and contexts when attempting to persuade historically marginalized audiences.

Because this book explores issues of tension between groups and organizations and quests for knowledge legitimation of a historically marginalized group, the case studies in this book were conducted using a cultural-studies approach (Longo, 1998, p. 54). Bernadette Longo provides a thorough discussion of technical communication and cultural theory in "An Approach for Applying Cultural Study Theory to Technical Writing Research" and describes ways that many technical communicators have fallen short of successful cultural-studies research because they studied discursive practices within an organization without examining how these practices affect or were affected by external groups (Longo, 1998, p. 57). Charlotte Thralls and Nancy Blyler assert that "it is not enough for the researcher to track networks of relationships *within* an organization, discipline, profession, institution, or industry; researchers must also track linkages with discourses and practices outside of these domains" (Thralls & Blyler, 1993, p. 190). As such, a cultural-studies perspective of regulatory writing would expand outside of the government agency to explore how external factors, like the participation or lack of participation of certain ethnic groups impact regulation invention. Longo also states, "choosing a coherent theoretical framework for a cultural study is crucial to understanding its results" (Longo, 1998, p. 62). As is often the case in technical communication and cultural studies, the theory that guided this research is borrowed from another discipline, intercultural communication; I used identity negotiation theory (Ting-Toomey, 1999, p. 25) as the theoretical framework for my study. In *Communicating Across Cultures,* Stella Ting-Toomey states, "the fundamental basis of the identity negotiation theory posits that individuals in all cultures desire to be competent communicators in a diverse range of interactive situations" (p. 27). Intercultural conflicts that impede this cultural competence include lack of trust-building skills that block intercultural negotiation (p. 222).

My cultural-studies approach to this project prohibited me from examining contemporary regulatory writing styles or invention without also considering how these rhetorical forces influence groups outside of the government agency. Since the Texas Black Codes were primarily focused on African American Texans and contract-based labor, my contemporary study concentrates on a similar group: black business owners in Texas. To tie the focus group study to the contextual inquiry study conducted at the Child Care Licensing Division of the Texas Department of Family and Protective Services, I asked the focus group members to examine discourse written by this agency. Thus, I used the focus group methodology to examine the responses of African American business owners to Child Care Licensing regulations and regulation development in general. "Focus group theory is based on the assumption that the interaction of members of a small group will facilitate the uncovering of ideas that probably wouldn't surface if individuals were asked separately about their thoughts, feelings, and beliefs" (MacNealy, 1999, p. 177). The discussion of regulations and regulation development in small groups composed of people of the same ethnic group creates an atmosphere that will flesh out beliefs, attitudes, and opinions about regulation development that would be perceived as too controversial to discuss in multicultural settings. MacNealy recommends that focus groups be composed of subjects who share some similar qualities; in this case, ethnicity and entrepreneurship are the characteristics that the participants have in common (p. 183). Another commonality, which I discovered after the focus group meeting, included the fact that half of the focus group members were graduates of historically black colleges in Texas.

Robert Johnson argues "we can begin to confront the problem of constructing a polis truly open to users, one that is egalitarian in its best sense, if we return to the problem of user knowledge and consider it as a knowledge of action" (1998, p. 64). The application of this user-centered methodology is appropriate in this study of regulation development, because regulation writing or rulemaking is by definition a user-centered undertaking; public participation in regulation development is required in law and statute. This blend of tasks-oriented (contextual inquiry) and user-centered (focus groups) instruments unveiled factors that encourage or discourage African American trust in regulatory negotiations. The findings of this study is synthesized into an invention heuristic that can be used as an apparatus that helps researchers identify conflicts that discourage historically marginalized groups from trusting either government regulations or those who enforce and write them. The selection of an ethnic group as the external link to the regulatory agency is an attempt to address a gap in technical communication literature with regard to intercultural communication within the United States. In "Multicultural Issues in Technical Communication,"

Emily Thrush, a technical communication scholar, whose research interests include international technical communication, discusses the growing number of ethnic minorities in workplaces in the United States, but concedes "it is hard to find in the literature any acknowledgement that we need to understand the processes to produce effective technical documents and training materials for workplaces that include members of subcultures. The need for research in this area is urgent" (1997, p. 173).

To mitigate the potential for researcher bias in my discourse analysis of Texas Black Codes, I enlisted another researcher to help code the various trust and distrust categories in my analysis of Texas Black Codes and measured the rate of interrater reliability (MacNealy, 1999, pp. 38, 58). In my focus group data, I solicited the help of a facilitator to reduce the possibility of leading questions or gestures in my interaction with focus group participants. I also used discourse analysis to analyze the results of my focus groups with African American business owners and my contextual inquiry study at a State of Texas agency. Still, with my attention to validity and reliability in my research, I was constantly challenged with the various limitations that we find in analyzing prose. Richard Lanham acknowledged these limitations in *Analyzing Prose* when he described the traditional stylistic choices in their conventional dichotomous extremes—noun and verb styles, parataxis and hypotaxis, periodic and running styles, voiced and unvoiced styles, high and low styles, and opaque and transparent styles. In this work, Lanham troubled long still waters, not by questioning the validity of styles such as the high and low styles, but suggesting that the reader demands a "transparent style" for understanding prose and nonfiction, while this same reader is in search of an "opaque style" to critique and analyze fiction and poetry (2003, p. 209). Years before beginning my examination of regulatory writing, I witnessed an example of Lanham's assessment in a poetry-writing seminar. As students enrolled in the seminar, our first assignment was to write a letter to our classmates informing them of types of language and poetry that we did not want to hear that semester. No one wanted to hear rhymes, plain language, or clichés. Most of my classmates thought that only a few poets used rhymes or clear language effectively in poetry and some even presumed that most of these poets were dead. The group reached consensus: veiled language in poetry would be a good starting point. Why did the poetry students prefer veiled language? The answer to this question might be because veiled language appeals to those readers who consider themselves to be higher-level thinkers or perform at the higher levels in Bloom's Taxonomy. Figures of speech and metaphors, whether in poetry or prose, allow many readers to use those higher-level thinking skills in Bloom's evaluation stage; in poetry and fiction, readers like to critique and evaluate. Poetry critics want more than comprehension and understanding; they want the challenge of solving a linguistic puzzle and critiquing the arrangement of its parts. Although it can be argued that some tropes clarify language, in some discourse, tropes give us just enough ambiguity to validate varying interpretations of the same words (Baake, 2003, pp. 2–3). Of poetry, Longinus wrote, "a certain mythical exaggeration is allowable, transcending altogether mere logical credence" (1952, p. 105) But in his examination of the appropriate uses of figures of speech in prose he argued, "the use of figures has a peculiar tendency to rouse a suspicion of dishonesty, and to create an impression of treachery, scheming, and false reasoning" (p. 108). Clearly, while students in my poetry-writing workshop craved veiled language, a similar style of writing would evoke distrust in a laborer or business person attempting to follow government rules and regulations.

Weeks later, in this same poetry seminar, the class read a poem with one line that was several words longer than the other lines in the stanza, creating a visual affect our professor called a "swinging affect." This particular line pulled the readers eyes beyond the rest of the text near the right margin. This visual effect was deemed "effective" because it accompanied the context of the line, a line of the poem that references a sudden shift from one extreme place to another. The unconventionally long line strengthened the poem because it made the students see the text. Lanham argues that those of us who study prose err by promoting a prose writing style, plain or complex, that helps us to look through text but not see it (2003, p. 79), while Carolyn Rude asserts, "In academia, the field of writing studies, including composition and technical communication, has expanded its focus in the past several years from text alone to the uses of the text. . . . A concept of delivery that extends beyond publication may help students and professional writers get to this understanding of the relationship of text to social action" (Rude, 2004, p. 284). Consequently, I assert that historically distrustful audiences will begin to both "see" and "use" regulatory text, through participation and compliance, not if we arrange the words on paper in an unconventional manner, but if we remove the veil. To begin this task, removing the veil from regulatory discourse, I recommend the practical application of the theoretical and evaluative tools applied in the rest of this book.

CHAPTER II

Case Study I–
Texas Black Codes of 1866:
Identifying Discourse Markers of Trust

In 1917, W. E. B. Dubois wrote and published an essay titled "Houston," in the NAACP's *The Crisis* magazine (Lewis, 1995, p. 448). The essay describes an incident where members of the Third Battalion of the Black Twenty-Fourth United States Infantry shot and killed white Houston police officers and civilians after a black soldier was arrested for interfering with a Houston police officer's arrest of a black woman in the Fourth Ward area of Houston, Texas (Haynes, 2003, p. 1; Lewis, 1995, p. 448). Texas, like many other southern states, has a long history of intergovernmental conflicts between the federal officials and militia and the state and local governments. In regulatory discourse, this history dates back 50 years prior to the Houston riot and is documented in the 11th Texas Legislature's laws or Texas Black Codes and in monthly reports and letters written by employees of the War Department's State of Texas Bureau of Refugees, Freedmen, and Abandoned Lands. Within these artifacts, the Texas Black Codes and Freedman's Bureau reports and letters, is documentation of the regulation of the labor of freed blacks (Moneyhon, 2003, p. 1). While the Black Codes attempted to legitimize a legal form of contract-endorsed servitude, the Freedman's Bureau reports, letters, and policy describe federal efforts to nullify inhumane and unfair contracts. The confusion that these conflicting laws and policy caused Texas blacks are clearly described in a letter from Freedmen's Bureau Brigadier General and Assistant Commissioner Edgar M. Gregory to Benjamin G. Harris, Esq. and Foreman Grand Jury of Panola County, Texas, dated January 25, 1866, when Gregory wrote, "it is but rational that those who live remote from the offices of our agents, not knowing whom to trust or what to believe, comprehending their relation but imperfectly as to their former masters but imperfect masters, will gain the knowledge of their rights and duties more slowly than those who live near the points of information and relief" (Gregory, 2002c). In this chapter, I conduct a rhetorical and historical analysis of Texas Black Codes enacted during the 1866 Texas' 11th Legislative Session in order to reveal that Texas regulations written during this period surely contributed to the "distrust" that Gregory mentions.

To support my analysis, I rely on Barry Crouch's historical accounts of the intergovernmental conflicts resulting from the Texas' 11th Legislature's promulgation of Texas Black Codes and the Texas Freedmen's Bureau's attempts to nullify the implementation of those codes. Crouch defines Texas Black Codes as "those series of laws passed by the states comprising the defeated Confederacy that applied directly or indirectly to African Americans" (1999, p. 263). Crouch suggests that the text of the codes intentionally avoided mention of race, but much of the content of the codes were indeed written to regulate the activities of blacks and were borrowed from the "harshest of codes from those that had been previously legislated by the five southern states," and the codes "maintained a nondiscriminatory façade that fooled no one" (p. 264). The bulk of the Texas codes promoted unfair labor contracts between white Texans and freed blacks, which provided little legal protection for employees or freedmen; vagrancy laws, which served as a means of forcing unemployed freed slaves into unfair employment contracts, and the worst of the codes—apprentice codes—that forced black children into "guardianships" with white Texans to serve as "a cheap source of labor" (p. 265).

Crouch makes it clear that even in these early years after the Emancipation Proclamation, there was a "black community" that protested to the Freedmen's Bureau regarding the injustices they suffered at the hands of white Texas "employers" or "guardians"; and in resistance to Texas Black Codes "Texas blacks endeavored to take care of their own and bring orphaned or so-called 'parentless' children into the confines of the black community" (Crouch, 1999, pp. 268, 271). Still, much of Crouch's argument is not to reveal the offenses of the Texas State Legislature, but to defend the actions of the Freedmen's Bureau, an agency that Crouch, like W. E. B. DuBois, viewed as a help to the freed slave (p. 278; DuBois, 1901, p. 362). An example of the Freedmen's Bureau's diligence is the counteracting of the efforts of legislators, sheriffs, and courts to indenture freed blacks through contracts and apprenticeships that freed slaves knew nothing about, because most of them could not read and had "no knowledge of the apprenticeship until after their consummation by the court" (Crouch, 1999, p. 273). According to Crouch, in such cases, Freedmen's Bureau staff invalidated these contracts. These events are but examples of the tenuous relationship between African Americans and government agencies. To explore the *ethos* of government agencies and whether these entities have ever evoked trust in the African American community, I will consult the works of scholars from a variety of disciplines, starting with Joel D. Aberbach and Jack L. Walker's attempt to define political trust in relation to race following the United States' Civil Rights movement.

IDENTIFYING DISCOURSE MARKERS OF TRUST

Joel D. Aberbach and Jack L. Walker attempted to define political trust in relation to race politics, and discuss the findings from their study, "Political Trust and Racial Ideology," which was conducted to measure political trust and race in Detroit, Michigan during the late 1960s. At the time of publication, 1970, there was very little scholarly material examining race and trust, but the concept of political trust was closely associated with "mutual respect" and "good faith" and defined as, "the evaluative orientation toward government" (pp. 1199, 1203). In conducting their study, the authors presented questionnaires to black and white citizens of Detroit in an attempt to measure varying orientations toward local and federal government, socioeconomic factors that might influence their orientation toward the government, and any correlations between their expectations of equal treatment and trust in the government (pp. 1204–1209). The results, gathered using quantitative methods, suggest that blacks were less trusting than whites of both local and federal governments (p. 1203), socioeconomic status was not an indicator in varying levels of trust between blacks and whites (p. 1205), white distrust of the government was mostly influenced by fears that "blacks receive special treatment and are given favors without deserving them," and "distrust among upper class blacks [did] not arise so much from actual or experienced discrimination than empathy for others in the black community who experience insults in a worse form" (p. 1206).

The results of this study suggest that the African American relationship with the government, as it relates to trust, had indeed evolved since Booker T. Washington's arguments regarding blacks' excessive dependance and trust in the government in the early part of the century; African Americans did not trust the government as much as white Americans (1901, p. 58). Aberbach and Walker stated, "black people are beginning to reject their traditional ties with paternalist friends and allies" (1970, p. 1204). In analyzing regulatory text to evaluate language that evokes trust or distrust between African Americans and government organizations, Aberbach and Walker's attention to "respect" and "good faith" are useful concepts to use as categories in a systematic study of language in regulations. Aberbach and Walker argue that political trust is largely determined by the political decisions made by government officials and the reactions these decisions provoke (p. 1202). Although this view takes the action of the government agency and the reaction of the citizen into consideration, it leaves out the impact that rhetoric may play in shaping a reaction. Arguably, reactions to public-policy decisions that are perceived as negatively impacting a group may be lessened if framed in a language that suggests mutual respect and good faith.

Almost 10 years after the Aberbach and Walker study, F. Glen Abney and John D. Hutcheson, Jr. continued the discussion of the relationship between race and political trust in another city with a large African American population:

Atlanta, Georgia. In "Race, Representation, and Trust: Changes in Attitudes After the Election of a Black Mayor," the authors used quantitative research methods to compare political trust levels in African American and white Americans in 1970 and 1976 (Abney & Hutcheson, 1981, p. 93). Both studies employed survey data and random sampling and selected participants who were citizens of Atlanta during both periods (p. 93). The major differences between the 2 years was the fact that in 1973, the citizens of Atlanta had elected their first black mayor; also during this period, the impeachment hearings of President Richard Nixon were held, and political trust had decreased throughout the entire nation (pp. 93–94). Abney and Hutcheson rely on the work of Aberbach and Walker to make the generalization that political distrust levels in large nonpartisan cities like Detroit and Atlanta vary only slightly from local governments to the Federal Government, and thus, the Watergate Affair did impact measurements of political trust in cities (Abney & Hutcheson, 1981, p. 94). Abney and Hutcheson's results indicated that African American trust in their local government remained almost the same during this period, whereas white Americans' trust in the government declined on a par with national trends (Abney & Hutcheson, 1981, p. 96.) Also, while the number of white Americans who believed that they received preferential treatment declined from 1970 to 1976, a number of blacks "perceived an increase in the equity of the city government's policies" (p. 98).

This study suggests that African Americans' distrust of the government is closely linked to their perception of the involvement of other African Americans in policy-making decisions. If, even during Watergate, African Americans' perception of equal treatment increased as a result of the presence of an African American mayor, there is quite possibly a positive correlation between African Americans' perception of participation in policy making and their trust in the government. The implications for such a correlation and regulatory writing might be that African American participation in regulation development may in turn increase trust in regulations. Another possibility is that the language used in regulations may not be as important as a perception of influence or participation in regulation development.

In 1988, Susan E. Howell and Deborah Fagan argued that Abney and Hutcheson's study is "the only research known to us that varies political reality" and suggests that Abney and Hutcheson's study failed to employ Center for Political Studies questions and were unable to "make the empirical link with the black mayor" (Howell & Fagan, 1988, p. 344). Howell and Fagan, using Center for Political Studies questions, examined yet another city with a large African American population, New Orleans, in an attempt to gauge African American trust levels in cities with black mayors (p. 344). New Orleans' citizens, 50% of whom were African American at the time of their study, were interviewed via telephone, and their responses suggests that "a black city administration changes black attitudes about their political position" (p. 345). The authors then asked two important questions: "If blacks are so responsive to the political environment, why aren't whites? Why are whites not distrusting in New Orleans under the black administration?" (p. 345). The authors looked to a 1984 study, "Racial Differences in Political Conceptualization" by Paul Hagner and John. E. Pierce for answers (Howell & Fagan, 1988, p. 346). Hagner and Pierce argued that the Civil Rights movement had caused blacks to form a strong group political identity that was not inherent in other ethnic groups or racial groups (Howell & Fagan, 1988, p. 346).

In recent years, much of the group political identity that Howell and Fagan stated emerged out of the Civil Rights movement has been closely linked to new rifts between this group and government organizations. During the 2000 presidential elections, many black Floridians felt betrayed by the state electoral system when errors in tallying votes in predominately black districts prompted ballot recounts and claims of black disenfranchisement resurfaced in the African American community nationwide. Six years later, in George W. Bush's September 15, 2005 Jackson Square speech regarding Hurricane Katrina, Bush confessed, "As all of us saw on television, there is also some deep, persistent poverty in this region as well. And that poverty has roots in a history of racial discrimination, which cut off generations from the opportunity of America. We have a duty to confront this poverty with bold action" (Bush, 2005, p. 1). As Bush acknowledged the roots of black poverty in New Orleans, many black New Orleanians who survived Hurricane Katrina voiced distrust in the Federal Emergency Management Agency (FEMA) and the Federal Government. They claimed that the levees did not break as a result of the rising waters ushered in by Hurricane Katrina but were purposely destroyed by the Federal Government to flood the 9th Ward, which was predominately African American, and protect the city's historical district, the French Quarter. Although there is no evidence to support current claims of intentional levee breaks, this conspiracy theory does, after all, have historical precedent. In 1927, there was an intentional levee break that African American New Orleanians, young and old, "remembered" and use as evidence to support their distrust.

> New Orleans watched the Mississippi Valley floodwaters nervously. On a single day in April the city had received 14 inches of rain, which put parts of it under more than six feet of water; the French Quarter had two feet. If a levee broke, the city would be doomed.
>
> Eventually, fearful townspeople prompted the governor to dynamite a levee south of town to relieve the pressure on New Orleans. The city was spared. Others in the state weren't so lucky. (Leopold, 2005, p. 1)

In August 2005, the city was not spared, nor were the people. The levees did break, and the Corps of Engineers' Hurricane Katrina report acknowledged that "the levees failed because they were built in a disjointed fashion using outdated data" (CBS/AP, 2006, p. 1). Lt. Gen. Carl Strock, the Corp's chief duly recognized, "Words alone will not restore trust in the Corps" (CBS/AP, 2006, p. 1). After the disaster, President Bush's reference to what "all of us saw on television" was mostly poor black people waiting days for food and water at the Ernest Memorial Convention Center and the New Orleans Superdome in dangerous and deplorable living conditions. While much public discourse after Hurricane Katrina focused on looting and fraudulent use of FEMA debit cards, distrust and disbelief in the government was another constant theme voiced in the media and by the public, many of whom argued that the Federal Government's efforts on behalf of wealthy or middle-class white Americans would not have been delayed for approximately a week as was the case during the aftermath of Hurricane Katrina. These recurring incidents of conflict between government organizations in America and the African American community have planted seeds of distrust, which were initially based on legitimate claims and that after years of maintenance have made fertile ground for conspiracy theories and even paranoia. At the local level, Mayor Ray Nagin, a black man who many New Orleanians accused of failing to properly evacuate the citizens, was reelected less than a year after Hurricane Katrina. While Nagin was elected by both black and whites, many of those who voted to reelect him were those same citizens who were not evacuated by the city of New Orleans and were still displaced in Houston, Texas, Baton Rouge, Louisiana, and throughout the country.

Howell and Fagan's findings, as well as the distrust of the African American community that followed Hurricane Katrina, give us reason to believe that a rhetorical analysis of the rhetoric in regulations and a study of systematic revisions on a sample group of the African American community might be twofold. First, there is a reason to believe that if rhetoric in regulations is shown to evoke distrust in a random sample of members of the African American community, well-informed generalizations can be made about the impact of these regulations on the whole group political identity (Howell & Fagan, 1988, p. 346). Second, the Hurricane Katrina disaster and its handling by the government might have effects on the relationship between African Americans and government agencies that do not exist between African Americans and black elected officials.

In an exploration of trust and distrust in other marginalized groups, outside of racial and ethnic politics, Trudy Glover argues that feminist theory interprets trust differently than contractual theory. Glover argues that in the early 1980s, during nuclear disarmament negotiations between the Soviet Union and Western countries, as a panelist and representative of Canadian antinuclear groups, she observed a rhetoric surrounding the issue of trust that sparked her examination of this subject and how it influenced negotiations between the groups (1992, p. 17). Glover argues, "When we trust others, we expect them to act in ways that are helpful, or at least not harmful to us" and she states, "trust affects the way we interpret what others do and say; it is in this sense a disposition" (p. 17). In that same vein, she suggests that when we distrust each other, we are more likely to interpret the actions of those we distrust in a negative way (p. 17). In a literature review of other feminist theorists' interpretation of trust, Glover examines contractual theory as defined by Annette Baier (p. 19). Baier argues that women "are painfully aware that relationships are not all voluntary, as contract theory would imply" (cited in Glover, 1992, p. 19). Glover suggests that contract theorists often ignore issues of trust and presume that negotiations are conducted in distanced relationships between "more or less free and equal adult strangers" (p. 19.)

Glover's interpretation of contractual theory as unrealistic because it downplays the role of trust in negotiations lends support to the argument that the *ethos* of the regulatory agency is negatively affected by regulatory language that does not evoke trust in regulated entities. Contractual theory, which is fundamentally an assertion that "a promise is legally enforceable if it is given as part of a bargain and it is unenforceable otherwise," considers only the *logos* of an exchange, not those emotional factors that are so important in establishing relationships between parties, especially parties who hold different levels of power (Cooter & Ulen, 1988, p. 214).

To support Glover's argument that extremist interpretations of negotiation theories are indeed unrealistic, Arthur M. Okun, in his book, *Equality and Efficiency: The Big Tradeoff,* argues that although "rights" are in some sense equivalent to deadweight loss, a civilized society will decide to make deliberative trade-offs between equality and economic efficiency in government interactions with its public (1975, pp. 6–8). To magnify his point, he presents two vastly different perspectives on the value of either equality or efficiency and explains how a government that subscribes to the ideals of one in lieu of the other would create negative relations between governments and citizens (p. 90). To represent extreme interpretations of equality, Okun brings John Rawls into the discussion. Okun quotes Rawls when he states, "John Rawls' difference principle, which insists that 'all social values . . . are to be distributed equally unless unequal distribution of any . . . is to everyone's advantage'—in particular, to the advantage of the typical person in the least-advantaged group" (p. 92). As an example of support for only efficiency, Okun quotes Milton Friedman, who posited, "Give priority to efficiency" (p. 92). Okun's response is that both equality and efficiency should be considered in policy making, and he suggests that the elementary concepts of economics will not suffice in the "real world"; he argues that trade-offs between equality and efficiency are never easy, but they are necessary (p. 90).

The arguments presented in Okun's book provide a framework for responses to anticipated questions about the costs and the value of examining regulations to uncover discourse that may promote distrust and in some way impact equality or even perceived equality of various audiences. Fortunately, the costs of conducting a rhetorical analysis to categorize language that may promote trust or distrust are not nearly as costly as continuing to develop regulations in a cultural vacuum.

Often, in collaborative writing processes such as regulation development, historically marginalized groups are distrustful processes because they believe their "voices" are not heard and that invention is indeed performed in a vacuum. Karen Burke LeFevre argues "many of us have indeed read 'autonomous themes' (and perhaps written them ourselves in English 101) in which the writer and the writing seem asocial, and invention appears to occur in a vacuum," but she goes on to argue that no invention is asocial (1987, p. 17). LeFevre argues that invention as a solitary act is a fiction perpetuated by composition theorists, who argue the existence of "a real voice" or creative writers inspired by the Romantic Tradition, who suggest that writers have an "inner voice" that they use to compose alone (pp. 17, 51). LeFevre argues that fallacy of an individual voice is influenced by both Platonic and capitalistic values that promote individual invention over collective or collaborative invention (pp. 17–19, 52). This view of invention, as collaborative, even if there is only one writer, suggests that there are external and internal influences in writing. LeFevre states, "If we extend the rhetorical invention, Michel Foucault's view of discourse, an endless potentiality that is occasionally evidenced in speech or writing, then we will study invention as a process extending over time, a process both enabled and manifested through talk and text" (p. 125).

Although the following discourse analysis focuses on the Texas Black Codes of 1866, a similar longitudinal study of regulatory writing, in a historical context, could unveil rhetorical devices used in regulations to embrace African Americans, Latinos, Native Americans, Asians, and women, especially as these regulations are amended, revised, translated, and repealed over the years. Also, a discourse analysis tracking the various rhetorical devices employed over a long period could disclose language patterns and rhetorical strategies that evoke not only trust or distrust but also reveal evolving characteristics of a government agency's collective voice, a voice that includes those who do not actively participate in regulation-development processes. If these patterns or rhetorical devices are discovered, they can be duplicated in conscious efforts to promote trust and goodwill between government agencies and regulated entities.

DISCOURSE ANALYSIS OF TEXAS BLACK CODES

In my analysis of the Texas Black Codes, I identified rhetorical choices that promoted discord and distrust in relationships between freed black Texans and state and local governments. The following codes were examined to see if trust or distrust would be evoked in audiences required to comply with these regulations:

- Chapter LXIII. An Act establishing General Apprentice Law and defining the obligations of Master and Mistress and Apprentice;
- Chapter LXXIII. An Act to amend an Act entitled an Act to adopt and establish a Penal Code for the State of Texas, approved August 28th, 1856, and to repeal portions thereof;

- Chapter LXXX. An Act Regulating Labor Contracts;
- Chapter LXXXII. An Act to provide for the punishment of persons tampering with, persuading or enticing away, harboring, feeding or secreting laborers or apprentices, or for employing laborers or apprentices under contract of service to other persons;
- Chapter CXI. An Act to define the offence of Vagrancy, and to provide for the punishment of Vagrants; and
- Chapter CXXVIII. An Act to define and declare the rights of persons lately known as Slaves, and Free Persons of Color.

I considered other documents that provide the historical and cultural contexts in which these regulations were written, implemented, and received. The primary audience for these regulations was made up of white citizens (landowners, courts, and law enforcement) and the secondary audience consisted of recently freed black slaves, an audience historically ignored. Viewing these artifacts from a cultural studies framework obligated me to examine the regulations from the perspective of the audience who had the least access to the documents, yet were the most affected by the text: recently freed black slaves. Barry A. Crouch's essay, "To Enslave the Rising Generation: The Freedman's Bureau and the Texas Black Code," which I discussed in the previous chapter, provided significant contextual data to facilitate a discourse analysis of Texas Black Codes (Crouch, 1999, pp. 261–287). The other text I examined for this purpose was James P. Butler's 12-page monthly report, which is handwritten on what appears to be a preformatted form. The purpose of the untitled form, which includes a printed statement suggesting that the form is "In compliance with Circular Letter, dated December 31, 1866," is to provide the federal Freedmen's Bureau officials reports of contractual conflicts between Texas' freedmen and whites and to report criminal offences involving or inflicted on freedmen (Butler, 1867, pp. 1–12). The monthly report examined in this study consists of a questionnaire that prompts Butler to provide handwritten responses to several questions regarding the conditions of freedmen or former slaves in his jurisdiction, Huntsville, Texas, and posed specific questions about the implementation of Texas Black Codes in the area. I found Butler's report while searching the National Archives Records of the Texas Bureau of Refugees, Freedman, and Abandoned Lands records from 1865 to 1870. Edgar M. Gregory's letters, report, and the policy circular were also transcribed from National Archives Records.

The Federal Government's Freedmen's Bureau's regulations were disseminated via circular letters or announcements, and it is obvious that James P. Butler's monthly report is in compliance with the circular letter referenced on the top of the form. Thus, circulars, letters, and reports that appear to be very similar to our contemporary policy memorandums provided bureau field staff with regulations for carrying out Freedmen's Bureau initiatives. One such regulation is outlined in a Freedmen's Bureau Circular dated October 17, 1865. This circular was written by Edgar M. Gregory 1 year before the promulgation of Texas Black Codes, but appears to respond to the same issue, the fair treatment of freed slaves in labor negotiations, contracts, and means of dealing with former slaves who become classified as vagrants (Butler, pp. 1–12). This circular, along with numerous letters and reports written by Gregory and Butler, provide the evidence that allows us to situate Texas Black Codes within their historical context.

To conduct an effective discourse analysis, I identified discourse markers for inferences about "persons involved [who] have long been dead" (MacNealy, 1999, p. 124). I found discourse markers of trust in the literature examined earlier in this chapter and in the work of Stella Sting Toomey, which I addressed in Chapter 1 of this book. The following discourse markers in Table 2.1, derived from these scholars' work, were used to code the text of Texas Black Codes into language that would likely evoke trust or distrust in recently freed black Texans.

FINDINGS OF DISCOURSE ANALYSIS

In 1866, DuBois' color line was ceremoniously unveiled in the Texas State Legislature's Black Codes and in the environment in which they were written and implemented. The writers, state legislators, wrote Black Codes "to frustrate Congress in its drive to provide legal equality for blacks" (Crouch, 1999, p. 262). After conducting a discourse analysis of these Black Codes, it is obvious that much of the language in these regulations was interpreted differently by legislators and their agents—courts and civil officers—and the Freedmen's Bureau. According to Barry A. Crouch, "before the [Texas] legislature enacted an apprenticing statute, the Texas [Freedmen's] Bureau, as a consequence of black persistence, adopted a four-point policy regarding indentures" (1999, p. 271). The four bureau regulations referenced by Crouch, like the six regulations listed in Edgar M. Gregory's October 17, 1865, policy circular, were written prior to the Black Codes and very likely in anticipation of them. Although much of the legislature's more accommodating language in the Black Codes is almost identical to language promulgated in the Freedmen's Bureau's policy circular, there are clear differences that either represents the legislature's blatant lack of regard for the Texas Freedmen's Bureau's regulations and its existence. The Freedmen's Bureau regulations in the October 17, 1865, policy circular include language that would indeed create the parameters for the creation of voluntary contracts between freedmen and whites and in doing so promote African American trust in government regulations and staff. On the contrary, the Texas Legislature's Black Codes, even in duplicating language used in the Freedmen's Bureau regulations, as well as the environment in which these laws were implemented, promoted punitive, binding, and involuntary contracts between white "masters" and "mistresses" and black subordinates. Edgar M. Gregory and James P. Butler's reports and letters provide the historical context for the

Table 2.1 Discourse Markers of Trust and Distrust

Discourse markers of trust	Discourse markers of distrust
Regulated parties are treated as equal adult strangers or with mutual respect (Aberbach & Walker, 1970, p. 1199; Glover, 1992, p. 19; Okun, 1975, pp. 90-92).	Regulated parties are not treated as equal adult strangers or with respect (Aberbach & Walker, 1970, p. 1199; Glover, 1992, p. 19; Okun, 1975, pp. 90-92).
All regulated parties have equal rights or responsibilities (Aberbach & Walker, 1970, p. 1204; Abney & Hutcheson, 1981, p. 97).	Overt discrimination against some regulated parties (Aberbach & Walker, 1970, p. 1204; Abney & Hutcheson, 1981, p. 97).
Regulations are enforced by credible arbitrators (Ting-Toomey, 1999, p. 223).	Regulations are enforced by arbitrators with questionable credibility (Ting-Toomey, 1999, p. 223).
Language used in regulations is consistent with actions in the enforcement of the regulations and promote good faith (Aberbach & Walker, 1970, p. 1199; Ting-Toomey, 1999, p. 223).	Language used in the regulations is inconsistent with actions in the enforcement of the regulations or intent of the regulations (Aberbach & Walker, 1970, p. 1199; Ting-Toomey, 1999, p. 223).
Fines are assessed fairly and help regulated parties (Glover, 1992, p. 17).	Fines and/or physical punishment are assessed disproportionately and harm regulated parties (Glover, 1992, p. 17).
Regulations promote voluntary labor contracts (Glover, 1992, p. 19).	Regulations promote involuntary labor contracts (Glover, 1992, p. 19).

Freedmen's Bureau regulations and speak to the agency's interpretations of the Black Codes.

The results of the discourse analysis of Texas Black Codes are listed in Table 2.2. The findings from the rhetorical and historical analysis of the Black Codes are overwhelmingly skewed toward language that would likely promote distrust in an African American audience. Of the 45 sections of Black Codes, 35 contained language that fit exclusively under the distrust categories, 7 include language that fit exclusively under the trust categories, and 3 did not fit in either category. Of the 35 sections that fit exclusively under distrust categories, 7 fit into two different distrust categories. Of the 7 sections that fit exclusively under trust categories, 2 sections fit into two different trust categories. Table 2.3 and Table 2.4 contain the actual text of the Texas Black Codes, the

Table 2.2 Identifying Language in Regulations that Evoke Black Trust or Distrust in Texas Black Codes

Discourse markers of trust	Number of occurrences	Discourse markers of distrust	Numbers of occurrences
Regulated parties are treated as equal adult strangers or with mutual respect (Aberbach & Walker, 1970, p. 1199; Glover, 1992, p. 19; Okun, 1975, pp. 90-92).	0	Regulated parties are not treated as equal adult strangers or with respect (Aberbach & Walker, 1970, p. 1199; Glover, 1992, p. 19; Okun, 1975, pp. 90-92.	6
All regulated parties have equal rights or responsibilities (Aberbach & Walker, 1970, p. 1204; Abney & Hutcheson, 1981, p. 97).	1	Overt discrimination against some regulated parties (Aberbach & Walker, 1970, p. 1204; Abney & Hutcheson, 1981, p. 97).	6
Regulations are enforced by credible arbitrators (Ting-Toomey, 1999, p. 223).	1	Regulations are enforced by arbitrators with questionable credibility (Ting-Toomey, 1999, p. 223).	10
Language used in regulations is consistent with with actions in the enforcement of the regulations and promote good faith (Aberbach & Walker, 1970, p. 119; Ting-Toomey, 1999, p. 223).	1	Language used in the regulations is inconsistent with actions in the enforcement of the regulations or intent of the regulations (Aberbach & Walker, 1970, p. 1199; Ting-Toomey, 1999, p. 223).	10
Fines are assessed fairly and help regulated parties (Glover, 1992, p. 17).	3	Fines and/or physical punishment are assessed disproportionately and harm regulated parties (Glover, 1992, p. 17).	7
Regulations promote voluntary labor contracts (Glover, 1992, p. 19).	2	Regulations promote involuntary labor contracts (Glover, 1992, p. 19).	2

historical context used to code the sections as text that would evoke trust or distrust, and the specific trust or distrust categories under which each section most appropriately fit. When analyzing Texas Black Codes in their historical contexts, "Language used in the regulations is inconsistent with actions in the enforcement of the regulations or intent of the regulations" was one of the most frequently coded categories (Aberbach & Walker, 1970, p. 1199; Ting-Toomey, 1999, p. 223). In Table 2.3, Chapter LXXX, Section 5 suggests that minors should be included as laborers. Although this section of the Black Codes is almost a duplicate of the language used in the October 17, 1865, circular distributed by the Freedmen's Bureau, the word "minors" was added by the Texas legislature. The October 17, 1865, circular states, "For Plantation Labor 1. Such contracts will be made with Heads of families. They will embrace all the Members of the family who are able to work" (Gregory, 2002e, p. 1). We know from the historical account of Barry A. Crouch that Texas citizens knew that "[on] the surface, the 1866 Texas black code appeared to ignore race, but it was designed to apply only to freedpeople" (1999, p. 264). Crouch suggests that the focus in the Black Codes on apprenticing minors was an attempt to "secure the labor of these black youngsters for a period of years" (p. 267). Thus, what appears to be a subtle change in the Black Codes to include the reference to "minors" was actually a maneuver to classify black minors as laborers and in turn make them vulnerable to the unfair labor contracts and apprenticeships, which were full of punitive clauses (11th Texas Legislature, 1866d, p. 995).

Evidence of another category used to code the language in Texas Black Codes, "Fines and/or physical punishment are assessed disproportionately and harm regulated parties" was apparent in several sections of the Texas Black Codes (Glover, 1992, p. 17). In Table 2.3, Chapter LXIII, Section 6 of the Black Codes suggests that apprentices, who were described in another section of this same chapter as "minors," were susceptible to corporal punishment. Also, the most lengthy section of the Texas Black Codes examined in this study, Chapter LXXX, An Act Regulating Labor Contracts, Section 9, explained punishments for "reasonable reductions of the laborers' wages," "negligent work, failure to obey employers, swearing in the presence of the employer or employer's family, leaving home without permission, and fighting" and sets out specific terms for laborers not to work on the Sabbath "except to take necessary care of stock and other property on the plantation, or to do necessary cooking or household duties, unless by special contract for work of necessity" (11th Texas Legislature, 1866d, p. 996). (Section 9 is obviously deceptive in that it suggests that laborers do not have to work on Sundays, but proceeds to list numerous duties that employers can request of laborers on this day.) Also, Chapter LXXX, An Act Regulating Labor Contracts, Section 7, states, "if any apprentice shall run away from, or leave the employ of his master or mistress without permission, said master or mistress may pursue and recapture said apprentice, and bring him before any Justice of the Peace of the county . . . in event of a refusal on the part

Table 2.3 Examples of Texas Black Codes that Evoke Distrust

Sections of black code	Historical context	Distrust category
CHAPTER LXXX. An Act Regulating Contracts for Labor. Section 1. Be it enacted by the Legislature of the State of Texas, That all persons desirous of engaging as laborers for a period of one year or less, may do so under the following regulations: All contract for labor for a longer period than one month shall be made in writing, and in the presence of a Justice of the Peace, County Judge, County Clerk, Notary Public, or two disinterested witnesses, in whose presence the contract shall be read to the laborers, and, when assented to, shall be signed in triplicate by both parties, and shall then be considered binding, for the time therein prescribed (11th Texas Legislature, 1866d, p. 994).	On Oct. 17th 1865, the Federal Government promulgated the following policy to sanction black labor contracts: I. All contracts with Freedmen for labor for the period of one Month and upwards must be conside [sic] to writing, Approved by an Agent of this Bureau [Freedmen's Bureau] and one Copy deposited with him in proper case he shall require security 33 (Gregory, 2002e, p.1). In a report to Lieutenant J. P. Richardson dated January 31, 1867, Freedmen's Bureau agent, James P. Butler wrote "Today a contract was brought to my notice, which the employer forced the freedpeople to sign. I disapproved the contract and informed the employer and the freedpeople" (Butler, p. 9).	Regulations are enforced by arbitrators with questionable credibility (Ting-Toomey, 1999 p. 223).
CHAPTER LXXX. An Act Regulating Contracts for Labor. Sec. 5. All labor contracts shall be made with the heads of families; they shall embrace the labor of all the members of the family named therein, able to work, and shall be binding on all minors of said families (11th Texas Legislature, 1866d, p. 995).	On Oct. 17th 1865, the Federal Government promulgated the following policy to sanction black labor contracts: II. For Plantation Labor 1. Such contracts will be made with Heads of families. They will embrace all the Members of the family who are able to work (Gregory, 2002e, p. 1). Note: Minors were not specifically mentioned in this federal policy. Barry Crouch wrote, "To make it even easier for whites to bind black children, the [Texas] legislature did not sanction black marriages" (Crouch, 1999, p. 265).	Language used in the regulations is inconsistent with actions in the enforcement of the regulations or intent of the regulations (Aberbach & Walker, 1970, p. 1199; Ting-Toomey, 1999, p. 223).

Table 2.3 (Cont'd.)

Sections of black code	Historical context	Distrust category
CHAPTER LXIII. An Act establishing a General Apprentice Law, and defining the obligations of Master and Mistress and Apprentice. Sec. 6. That in the management and control of an apprentice, the master or mistress shall have power to inflict such moderate corporeal chastisement as may be necessary and proper (11th Texas Legislature, 1866d, p. 980).	"One agent in Sterling encountered a youngster, previously apprenticed by the county court, who had obviously received 'harsh treatment.' The Bureau agent believed that the young man (no age given) was old enough to work for more than provisions and clothes and should be compensated for his labor. The Bureau agent refused to release the boy to the planter until the contract was signed, with the agent as the guardian, which entitled the minor to earnings" (Crouch, 1999, p. 271).	Fines and/or physical punishment are assessed disproportionately and harm regulated parties (Glover, 1992, p. 17).
CHAPTER LXIII. An Act establishing a General Apprentice Law, and defining the obligations of Master and Mistress and Apprentice. Sec. 12. The County Judge shall have power to hear and determine and grant all orders and decrees, as herein provided, as well in vacation as in term time; Provided, That, in all applications for apprenticeship, ten days' public notice, as in case of guardianship, shall be given, and no minor shall be apprenticed except at a regular term of said Court. Approved October 27, 1866 (11th Texas Legislature, 1866d, p. 981).	One field officer, Gary Barrett, wrote, "as it only requires a notification in the papers of the intention to indenture, and as very few freedpeople can read, those interested immediately have not knowledge of the apprenticeship until after its consummation by the Court" (Crouch 1999, p. 273).	Regulations are enforced by arbitrators with questionable credibility (Ting-Toomey, 1999, p. 223).

Table 2.4 Examples of Texas Black Codes that Evoke Trust

Sections of black code	Historical context	Trust category
CHAPTER LXXX. An Act Regulating Contracts for Labor. Sec. 2. Every laborer shall have full and perfect liberty to choose his or her employer, but when once chosen, they shall not be allowed to leave their place of employment, under the fulfillment of their contract, unless by consent of their employer, or on account of harsh treatment or breach of contract on the part of the employer, and if they do so leave without cause or permission, they shall forfeit all wages earned to the time of abandonment (11th Texas Legislature, 1866d, pp. 994–995).	In a letter from Brig. Gen. and Assistant Comm. E. M. Gregory to O.O. Howard dated January 31, 1866, Howard wrote, "The blacks were willing to work asking only that the promises made them by the planters be enforced by the Government. Under these conditions contracts were made freely with the freedmen and approved by the Bureau on liberal terms. There is a great variety of contracts between them and their employers and much vagueness of terms" (Gregory, 2002b, p. 1).	Regulations promote voluntary labor contracts (Glover, 1992, p. 19).
CHAPTER LXXX. An Act Regulating Contracts for Labor. Sec. 4. The Clerk of the County Court shall enter, in a well bound book kept for that purpose, a regular and alphabetical index to the contracts filed, showing the name of the employer, and the employed, the date of filing, and the duration of the contract, which book, together with the contract filed, shall, at all times, be subject to the examination of every person interested, without fee. The Clerk shall be entitled to demand from the party filing such contract, a fee of twenty-five cents, which shall be full compensation of all services required under this Act (11th Texas Legislature, 1866d, p. 995).	In a letter from Brig. Gen. and Assistant Comm E. M. Gregory to Gen. O.O. Howard dated April 18, 1866, Gregory wrote, "[I]n this State the rate of wages has not been fixed either as to Maximum or Minimum by any regulations from this Office. The only conditions required being that the laborer should perfectly understand what he was called upon to do. If the contract was not unfair, if the Negro understood it, and gave consent, it was enough" (Gregory, 2002a p. 2).	All regulated parties have equal rights or responsibilities (Aberbach & Walker, 1970, p. 1204; Abney & Hutcheson, 1981, p. 97).

Table 2.4 (Cont'd.)

Sections of black code	Historical context	Trust category
CHAPTER LXXX. An Act Regulating Contracts for Labor.Sec. 6. Wages due, under labor contracts, shall be a lien upon one-half of the crops, second only to liens for rent, and not more than one-half of the crops shall be removed from the plantation, until such wages are fully paid (11th Texas Legislature, 1866d, p. 995).	On Oct 17, 1865, the Federal Government promulgated the following policy to sanction black labor contracts: 33. II. For Plantation Labor 3. Such contracts will be a lien upon the Crop of which not more than one half will [be] removed untill [sic] all payments have been made, and untill [sic] the contract shall have been released by an Agent of this Bureau or Justice of the Peace in case it is impractable [sic] to procure the Services of Such Agents (Gregory, 2002e, p. 1). On January 31, 1866, Gregory wrote, "In many instances, instead of wages, a portion of the crop ranging from ¼ to ½ according to the special conditions of each case is pledged to the laborers and the instances are not infrequent where in addition to high percentage of the expected crop, the planter boards and lodges his workmen gratis" (Gregory, 2002b, p. 1).	Language used in regulations is consistent with actions in the enforcement of the regulations and promote good faith (Aberbach & Walker, 1970, p. 1199; Ting-Toomey, 1999, p. 223).
CHAPTER LXXX. An Act Regulating Contracts for Labor. Sec. 7. All employers, wilfully failing to comply with their contract, shall, upon conviction, be fined an amount double that due the laborer, recoverable before any court of competent jurisdiction, to be paid to the laborer; and any inhumanity, cruelty, or neglect of duty, on the part of the employer, shall be summarily punished by fines, within the discretion of the court, to be paid to the injured party; provided, that this shall not be so construed as a remission of any penalty, now inflicted by law, for like offences (11th Texas Legislature, 1866d, p. 995).	On Oct 17, 1865, the Federal Government promulgated the following policy to sanction black labor contracts: III. The usual remedies for Violation of Contract to the employer of forfeiture of Wages due and to the Freedman of damages Secured by lien or personal Security are assumed to be sufficient and all that practable [sic]" (Gregory, 2002e, p. 1).	Fines are assessed fairly and help regulated parties (Glover, 1992, p. 17).

of said apprentice to return, then the Justice shall commit said apprentice to the county jail" (p. 980). While sections of the Black Codes that were directly addressed to black laborers and apprentices are reminiscent and undoubtedly influenced by laws enacted and enforced during slavery, the only means of punishment directed at white employers are monetary fines, not physical punishment or incarceration (p. 995).

There is evidence that some white men, namely Freedmen's Bureau Agent James P. Butler, also suffered the threat of fines and physical punishment by county sheriffs, court officials, and civil officers who were responsible for enforcing the Black Codes. In Butler's report, he wrote, "The complainant was haping [sic] along the Public Square of Huntsville, when Burgess, in broad daylight ipsued [sic] out of the store, presented a derringer, loaded, cocked at complainant's heart, and bid him, 'if he had anything to say, to say it quick, for in one minute he was to be a dead man'" (Butler, p. 2). Butler identified himself as the complainant and Burgess as the county sheriff and wrote, "I consider it hardly worth repeating, is the removal of the present set of civil officers" (Butler, pp. 1-12). If James P. Butler, a white federal official, suffered such abuses by the local authorities, it is not likely that freed blacks could trust these same Texas officials as credible arbitrators of state laws. In Table 2.3, Chapter LXXX, Section 1, under "Historical context," Butler reports one incident where "the employer forced the freedpeople to sign" a labor contract, and Butler voided the contract (Butler, p. 9). Thus, Butler and other agents of the Freedmen's Bureau were helpful in protecting the rights of freed blacks, making good-faith efforts on their behalf, ensuring that their labor contracts were voluntary and not as discriminatory as the Texas Black Codes would allow, and offering help in lieu of punishment. In spite of this help from the Freedmen's Bureau staff, many recently freed blacks placed their trust in white landowners and contracted with them under the authority of the Texas Black Codes, and there is historical evidence to support this trust. Table 2.4 lists examples of ways the 11th Texas Legislature used language to promote trust that assured freed slaves that the State of Texas, not the Freedmen's Bureau, would protect their rights in contracted negotiations and apprenticeships with white landowners.

Of the eight Texas Black Codes placed in trust categories, three sections were related to the assessment of fines and punishment against white landowners or "planters" who failed to meet the demands agreed to in labor contracts. Although there is little evidence to support the collection of these fines by the State of Texas officials, there is evidence that black laborers entered into labor contracts with white landowners frequently and freely. Also, the codes listed in Tables 2.3 and Table 2.4 suggest that the Texas Legislature used the October 17, 1865, Freedmen's Bureau Circular as a model for some labor contract negotiations, but intentionally left this federal agency out of the contract approval process (Gregory, 2002e, p. 1). Under "Sections of Texas Black Code" in Table 2.3, notice that Chapter LXXX, Section 1 (11th Texas Legislature, 1866d, pp. 994-997) and the historical context from the Freedmen's Bureau Circular dated October 17, 1865 (Gregory, 2002e, p. 1), contain almost identical language and intent, but Texas legislators replace the duties of Freedmen's Bureau agents with county officials. Even with this apparent maneuver to lessen the Federal Government's influence on labor negotiations between blacks and whites in Texas, the Black Codes and historical context provided in Table 2.4 provide some evidence that some labor contracts were useful and some conflicts in contract negotiations between black laborers and white landowners were resolved with intervention by Freedmen's Bureau staff. Clearly, in the years following Reconstruction, these labor contracts, many of which were indeed unfair, finally allowed Texas black laborers to move from a slave status to sharecroppers.

The primary audience for the 11th Texas State Legislature's Black Codes of 1866 included recently freed black slaves, landowners who demanded the continuation of black labor, and county sheriffs and court officials who were willing to enforce these regulations, which were in violation of federal law (Crouch, 1999, pp. 262-271). During this time, it is fair to say that the recently freed blacks had no voice in regulatory matters because they were not citizens of the United States. Since there is little written record of the former slave's responses to these regulations, efforts to reconstruct or trace a history from these perceptions to the present day is not possible. What is possible is an examination of a period where federal regulations contradicted state regulations; this was a period of conflicts or what Foucault would call "discontinuity" or "the threshold of a function, the instant at which a circular causality breaks down" (Foucault, 1972, p. 9). The results of this study in conflict and discontinuity revealed that issues related to "truth" in regulations were gone. Texas Black Codes contained language that would evoke distrust in African American audiences because the content or *logos* of Texas Black Codes were "false," and the character or ethos of those who promulgated the regulations were compromised by federal agents who informed freed blacks of their rights to have contracts signed under Texas Black Codes voided. This analysis was not an attempt to discover the truth of the document but to reconstruct a rational audience's reaction to a state government's lack of *ethos,* the emotion (distrust) evoked by the enforcement of the wrong regulations, and this audience's response to fallacious arguments presented by the 11th Texas Legislature, all of which would certainly evoke distrust in rational audiences (Foucault, 1972, p. 6). The disenfranchisement of freed blacks in this country was an intentional breakdown in communication and governance; similar government-initiated ruptures have occurred throughout history with people of various ethnic, political, and socioeconomic backgrounds. In the next chapter, I examine the residuals of this type of "threshold, rupture, break, mutation, and transformation," and how, even if partially rectified with Plain English regulations, continued to contribute to conflicts between the law and reality for black laborers (Foucault, 1972, p. 5).

CHAPTER III

Texas Laws and Tacit Laws: Redefining Black Labor from "The Nadir" to Civil Rights

While Crouch (1999, p. 266), asserts that Texas Black Codes were repealed by the Texas Legislature during Reconstruction in 1870, historian Quintard Taylor explains, "Despite a Republican majority, Texas's first interracial legislature failed to repeal the black codes. Moderate Republicans joined Democrats to maintain most contract labor provisions, the convict labor system, the vagrancy statue, and the child apprenticeship law. Practically, however, these laws became moot as planter and freedpeople increasingly adopted sharecropping, thus eliminating the landowners' need to 'control' black labor" (Taylor, 1998, p. 111). In a sense, both Crouch and Taylor are correct in that the Black Codes, as they were in 1866, were not repealed during the 12th Legislative Session in 1870 but were repealed in the 1st Session of 1871, also part of the State of Texas' 12th Legislative Session (12th Legislature of State of Texas, 1871, pp. 90–91). Although the repeal of the Texas Black Codes took less than a full page of text, the implications of these repeals and the Freedman's Bureau's efforts toward this aim were significant in reshaping black labor, literacy, and migration. In this chapter, I demonstrate how various genres of technical communication, including regulations, manuals, and pamphlets, were used to help redefine post-Reconstruction labor and livelihood for black Texans.

It was during this period following Reconstruction, 1877–1901, that African Americans experienced what historian Rayford Logan (1954) coined "the nadir," or the lowest point in the lives of African Americans, where the hope that followed slavery was replaced with "constitutional disenfranchisement, physical and character assaults, and the proliferation of segregation laws" (Alford, 2003). One of the most notable and quite possibly the most effective civil rights advocate in post-Reconstruction years was Ida B. Wells, who wrote and published pamphlets that presented arguments against lynching in the South. Wells' pamphlets report technical data and statistics, include both text and visuals to communicate the severity of the problem, and inform her audience about health and safety (life and death) problems confronting the black community in the South. The scope and intent of Wells' pamphlets were to inform black and white America of the very present danger that the black community grappled with at the time.

Wells' pamphlets represent a form of technical communication addressing any audience (black or white) concerned enough to read and digest the macabre stories and statistics about lynchings in the South. While we know that Wells' work was influential in alerting Americans in the North and even an international audience about lynching in the South, there were no apparent rhetorical moves in her work to ignore the African American audience, which became increasingly literate during Reconstruction. There is certainly evidence to support the fact that Wells wrote directly for an African American audience in that, in addition to her pamphlets, she wrote, "editorials that encouraged African Americans in Memphis to leave a city that offered no protection of their rights of citizenship" (Royster, 1997, p. 4). Wells' crusade against lynching began as a very personal one after two black businessmen in Memphis, close friends of Ida B. Wells, were lynched because their grocery store was successfully competing against a white grocery store in close proximity (Royster, 1997, p. 2). Wells believed that there was a close link between lynching and economics and wrote that the lynchings of her two friends, "opened my eyes to what lynching really was. An excuse to get rid of Negros who were acquiring wealth and property and thus keep the race terrorized (quoted in Royster, 1997, p. 4). Successful freedmen turned business owners lived in cities throughout the South, including "Webster Wallace, former slave and later homesteader, [who] became one of the largest cattle ranchers in Texas, owning 10,000 acres of pastureland" (Thomas, 2000, p. 13). While lynching was an attack on blacks attempting to acquire wealth and property, sharecropping was a practice that would make certain that many never would. For the black laborer, sharecropping was the practice of renting a percentage of a farmer's land, farming it, and receiving a very small percentage of the proceeds of the sale of the harvest. While Wells and other civil rights activists spoke and wrote to international audiences in an effort to improve the conditions of blacks in the South, most black Texans continued to work as sharecroppers until the late 1930s. During this same period, the literacy rates for black Texans increased at rates unmatched in other states. "In 1900 black Texans recorded the lowest illiteracy rate in the South, 38 percent, and led in the number of high schools with nineteen" (Barr, 1996, p. 156) and by 1930 the illiteracy rate among Texas blacks was only 13% (p. 159). Black Texas sharecroppers as well as their employers needed to comply with laws containing instructions for handling the production of cotton and read and agree to the terms of farm lease contracts as shown in Figure 3.1.

To illustrate some of the work processes involved in sharecropping or farm leasing, I interviewed the daughter of Arthur Lee, a black Texas sharecropper who farmed land in Fort Bend County, Texas. During the 1920s and 1930s, Lee, a literate black Texan worked as a "straw boss" and sharecropper on land owned by a white Fort Bend County family, and Lee was one black man responsible for understanding and applying Texas' cotton laws. Lee's job was to manage or "oversee" laborers during the time of reaping the harvest; black and Hispanic laborers would travel to Fort Bend County and live in barns when picking cotton. His daughter, 83-year-old Nora Lee Williams of Houston, Texas recalls,

> My father was responsible for making sure that the laborers harvested the land, planted the cotton, and when the cotton got too thick, they would cut some of the cotton out, about a foot, so it wouldn't come up too thick. When the cotton came up—there were green bows as big as your fist, and when it ripened, those bows would open up and the white cotton would be in the bows. At that point, landowners would get help from Mexican [American] laborers from Laredo, Texas and from Mexico and some black laborers from other parts of the state. A lot of them would live in the barns behind our place. They'd put the long sacks on their shoulders and, as they picked, put the cotton in the sacks. Laborers and the straw boss were supposed to receive money for whatever amount of cotton they picked. Daddy and my brothers would take the cotton to a cotton gin in Richmond, Texas and the gin would separate the seeds from the cotton and put the cotton into bales. One season, I remember Daddy and my brothers harvested 12 bales of cotton, but the laborers were only paid for one bale—the rest went to the land owner. In the meantime, my daddy took care of the mules that pulled the wagons, the wagons, and harnesses; all of it was needed transport cotton. (personal interview, September 1, 2007)

Bankers in states throughout the country, including Texas, published user-friendly booklets for local farmers, businessmen and mechanics that listed laws and regulations that applied specifically to persons like Lee, who were responsible for baling and transporting cotton, as well as example contracts to be used by sharecroppers and land owners. In the preface of the 1906 edition of *Texas Laws Made Plain: Laws and Forms Prepared for Farmers Mechanics and Business Men,* D. E. Simmons, United States Attorney, Southern District of Texas wrote, "This book is not intended for the use of lawyers, but it is prepared that the general reader may have a fairly accurate [?] of most of our statutory law . . . I think will prove of interest to the farmer, stockman, mechanic and others who have not the time to make a special study of our laws. (Simmons & Simmons, 1906, Preface). Also in the front matter of the 1906 version of the manual, there is an insert from the AMERICAN NATIONAL BANK of Austin, Texas titled, "TO OUR FRIENDS," which reads,

> This compilation is intended for the use of those who desire to have at hand some convenient means of references in the general laws of Texas, without being compelled to resort to the bulky volume of our revised statutes, or to the numerous acts of the legislature. The work is not an abridgement of all

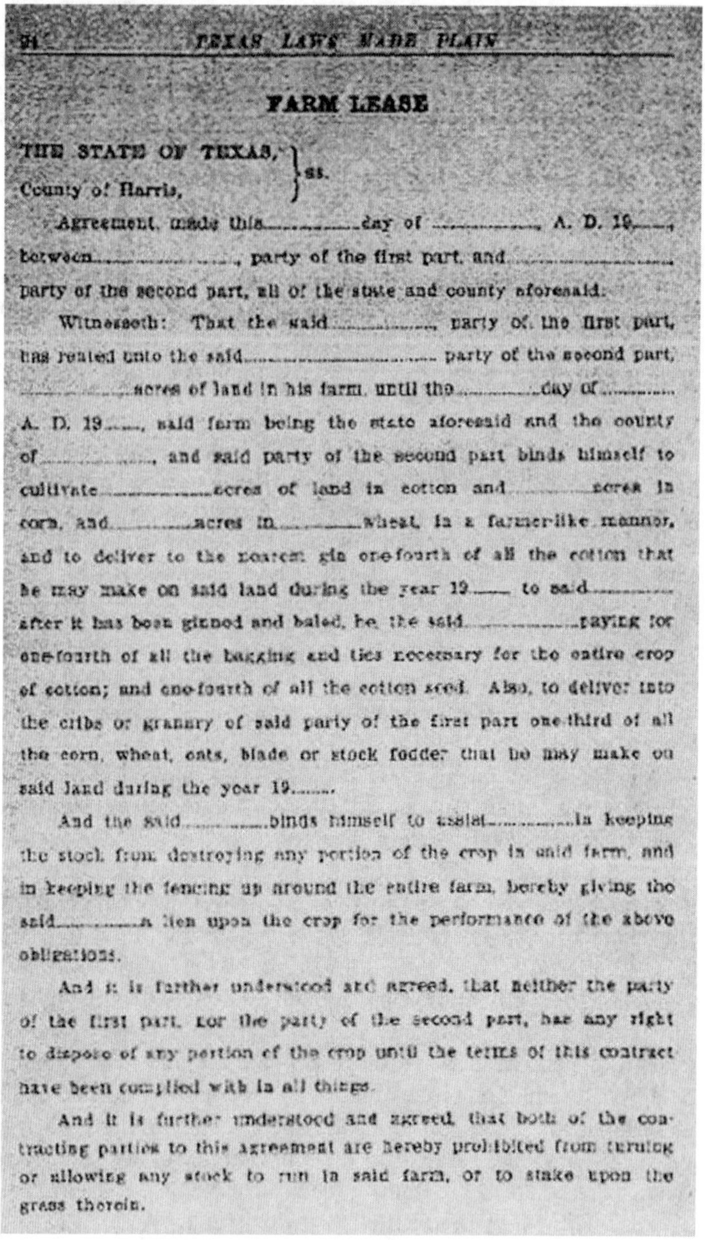

FARM LEASE

THE STATE OF TEXAS, } ss.
County of Harris,

Agreement, made this _____ day of _____, A. D. 19____, between _____, party of the first part, and _____ party of the second part, all of the state and county aforesaid:

Witnesseth: That the said _____, party of the first part, has rented unto the said _____ party of the second part, _____ acres of land in his farm, until the _____ day of _____ A. D. 19____, said farm being the state aforesaid and the county of _____, and said party of the second part binds himself to cultivate _____ acres of land in cotton and _____ acres in corn, and _____ acres in _____ wheat, in a farmer-like manner, and to deliver to the nearest gin one-fourth of all the cotton that he may make on said land during the year 19____ to said _____ after it has been ginned and baled, he the said _____ paying for one-fourth of all the bagging and ties necessary for the entire crop of cotton; and one-fourth of all the cotton seed. Also, to deliver into the cribs or granary of said party of the first part one-third of all the corn, wheat, oats, blade or stock fodder that he may make on said land during the year 19_____.

And the said _____ binds himself to assist _____ in keeping the stock from destroying any portion of the crop in said farm, and in keeping the fencing up around the entire farm, hereby giving the said _____ a lien upon the crop for the performance of the above obligations.

And it is further understood and agreed, that neither the party of the first part, nor the party of the second part, has any right to dispose of any portion of the crop until the terms of this contract have been complied with in all things.

And it is further understood and agreed, that both of the contracting parties to this agreement are hereby prohibited from turning or allowing any stock to run in said farm, or to stake upon the grass therein.

Figure 3.1. Form Lease Contract Form.
Source: *Texas Laws Made Plain*, 1921.

> **TEXAS LAWS MADE PLAIN**
>
> And it is further understood and agreed, that the said .... party of the second part, hereby agrees and binds himself to use due diligence in preventing the destruction of the houses and fences by fire or any other means, and to turn over the said houses and fences in the same good order and condition that they are at present on the ....day of................ A. D. 19.......
>
> It is further understood and agreed by the above mentioned contracting parties, that if the said party of the second part sows any small grain upon the above mentioned land, that the said party of the second part, shall, at his own expense, break up the stubble before the first day of................19......, and in default of same, party of the first part may do or have the same done at the expense of said party of the second part. It is further agreed that, in addition to the liens already provided, or to be provided by law, said party of the first part, is hereby fully empowered to take into his possession and sell, at the current market price, the first products of said crops as fast as the same can be prepared for market, to an amount sufficient to repay all advances made by said party of the first part, to said party of the second part, and to pay all rents, due, or to become due, on said land.
>
> In testimony of all the above, we hereunto sign our hands this ....day of............., A. D. 19......, in the presence of the witnesses signing below.
>
> Witnesses:

Figure 3.1. (Cont'd.)

of the laws of the state, but a compilation of those provisions of the statutes believed to be of most concern to the people in general. Such topics as arise in the every-day lives of our citizens are discussed by Hon. D. E. Simmons, who for five years was the assistant attorney general of the state of Texas, of the law firm of Rogan & Simmons, Austin, Texas. These topics are clothed in plain language, and can be understood by those who are not lawyers. This work has been prepared at large expense, and we present it to our friends, believing that it will give them a fair knowledge of the laws of our commonwealth, and after a careful reading of the same will prize it as a souvenir of no little value, and one that can be consulted with pleasure and profit for many years to come. (Simmons & Simmons, 1906, Preface)

The purpose of the *Texas Laws Made Plain* editions were to provide easy access to those instructional laws, many of which were labor laws applicable to Lee and other black Texas sharecroppers. Such laws would have included those concerning the correct procedure for bailing cotton, as enacted in 1911 by the Texas Legislature and excerpted from the *Texas Laws Relating to Labor of 1923*.

Section 111. Baling of Cotton Regulated; Penalty.

Every person, firm, corporation, or association of persons, owning or operating a compress in this State, and their agents and employees, are hereby required, in compressing, recompressing, baling or rebaling cotton bales, to so bind and tie every bale of cotton by them compressed, recompressed, baled or rebaled, that no such bale shall be delivered to any railroad company, or other common carrier, by such person, firm, corporation or association or persons, their agents or employees, unless such bale of cotton shall be free from all or any dangerously exposed ends of bands or buckles, or any dangerously exposed or protruding part of the ties, bands, buckles or splices used in tying or binding such bale of cotton. And any such person, firm, corporation or association or persons, who shall fail to bind or tie any bale of cotton by them compressed, recompressed, baled or rebaled, in the manner above provided, and shall deliver, or cause to be delivered, any such bale of cotton, to any railroad company, or other common carrier, such person, firm, corporation or association of persons, shall forfeit and pay to the State of Texas the sum of not less than $50, nor more than $250, which may be recovered in a civil suit brought in the name of the State of Texas in a court of competent jurisdiction. [R. C. S., 1911, Art. 1322.]

Section 112. Person, firm, etc., receiving for storage, transportation, etc., cotton not baled as required, liable for injuries to employee; duty of inspection.

Any person, firm, corporation or association of persons, receiving for storage, loading or transportation, or transporting, any such compress bale or bales of cotton, in this State, containing any dangerously exposed ends of bands or buckles, or any dangerously protruding part or parts of the ties, bands, buckles, or splices used in tying or binding such bale or bales of cotton, shall be liable in damages for injury to any person in the employ of such person, firm, corporation or association of persons, occasioned by reason of such dangerously exposed ends of bands or buckles or any dangerously exposed or protruding part or parts of the ties, bands, buckles or splices used in tying or binding such bale or bales of cotton, while in the discharge of the duties of such employment. The duty of inspection of such bales of cotton shall be on the employer and not on the employee. [*Id.*, Art. 1323] (Bureau of Labor Statistics, 1923, pp. 75–76)

Hon. D.E. Simmons and D. A. Simmons' plain language version of the same sections of the aforementioned law found in the *Texas Laws Made Plain* manual published in 1921 reads:

> **COTTON**
>
> **BALING REGULATED**—All persons owning or operating a compress are required to so compress or recompress cotton bales as to leave no jagged ends exposed or protruding; a violation subjecting the party to a penalty of not less than $50 nor more than $200 such amount to be recovered in a civil suit in the name of the State of Texas and paid to the state. (Simmons and Simmons, 1921, p. 23)
>
> **LIABILITY OF STORAGE COMPANIES**—Any person receiving for storage, loading for transportation, or transporting such compressed cotton with dangerously exposed ends or bands or buckles shall be liable in damages for injury to any person in the employ of the above parties handling such cotton, while in the discharge of the duties of such employment.
> The duties of inspection of such bales of cotton shall be on the employer and not on the employee. (Simmons and Simmons, 1921, p. 23)

To revise Section 111 into plain language, former Texas Attorney General D. E. Simmons and Assistant U.S. Attorney D. A. Simmons replaced the lengthy phrase, "Every person, firm, corporation, or association of persons, owning or operating a compress in this State, and their agents and employees" with "All persons owning or operating a compress," and in doing so, concisely communicated that anyone owning or operating a compress was required to use it in a certain way. Also in the first sentence of Section 111, the authors revised the lengthy, repetitive prepositional phrases, including "in compressing, recompressing, baling or rebaling cotton bales" and "by them compressed, recompressed, baled or rebaled." These prepositional phrases are redundant and include obvious information that the authors delete entirely. Also, while the lengthy codified version of Section 111 required the excessive use of commas that have proven to cause confusion in legal discourse, the concise plain language version includes one semicolon and one period. During the same period that the 1921 version of the cotton baling and storage laws were published, T. A. Rickard published the second edition of *Technical Writing*. In it, Rickard observed that lawyers avoided punctuation marks because incorrectly placed punctuation led to confusion (Rickard, 1920, 1923, pp. 306–307.) Notice that "shall" is used in both the legalese and plain language versions of Section 111. In reference to the "shall" versus "will" debate often associated with legal writing, Rickard wrote, "Originally 'shall' and 'will' were the present tenses of two verbs; 'should' and 'would' were their pasts; one of them had the meaning of command or obligation; and the other, of wish." During this period, "shall" is followed by something that the regulated party is obligated to do and "will" precedes a proposal or option; this explains the use of "shall" in plain language and legalese. In analyzing D. E. and D. A. Simmons' revision strategies, which included conciseness, deletion of unnecessary prepositional phrases, little punctuation, and avoidance of superfluous phrases, it is obvious that the Simmonses agreed with many of the tenants presented in Rickard's textbook on technical writing. Unfortunately, the *Texas Laws Made Plain* manuals failed to meet the ethical standards of honesty and accuracy in technical communication. In the next section of this chapter, I discuss inconsistencies between the intent and content in *Texas Laws Made Plain* and the Texas regulations in effect in 1906 and 1921. I also discuss inconsistencies between Texas regulations and societal laws from post-Reconstruction to the Civil Rights Era.

REDEFINING APPRENTICESHIP AND CONTRACT LABOR

While current definitions of apprenticeship describe a voluntary period that an individual who agrees, possibly under contract, to learn a new trade under the direction of someone who has already mastered the trade, the "apprenticeship" in the *Texas Laws Made Plain* manuals published in 1906 and 1921 is still defined as someone bound to work until the age of 21 (Simmons & Simmons, 1906, pp. 5–6).

APPRENTICES

> The county court may bind a minor as an apprentice, (1) when such a minor is an orphan without sufficient estate for his support and education; (2) when his parents have allowed him to become a charge of the county; (3) when his parents, by writing signed, filed and entered in the court consent to such apprenticeship. The duration of the apprenticeship shall be in the case of a male until he arrives at the age of twenty-one; and in the case of a female until she arrives at the age of eighteen or until she marries in the event she marries before that age.

On the cover of the 1921 *Texas Laws Made Plain* manual, the authors state the manual was "revised to include laws passed during the regular session legislature 1921" (Simmons and Simmons, 1921, Cover). This updated version of the manual included the following plain language version of the apprenticeship laws:

> **WHO MAY BE APPRENTICED**—The county court has jurisdiction over minors in the matter of apprenticeship, just as such court has jurisdiction in the matter of guardianships. The county court may bind a minor as an apprentice: (1) when the minor is an orphan and without sufficient estate for his maintenance and education; 2) when the parents have allowed him to become a charge upon the country; 3) when his parents, by writing signed, filed and entered of record in the court, consent to such apprenticeship. A

minor can be apprenticed only in the country of his residence (and after ten days in such county) and at a regular term of the court after ten days' notice as in the case of guardianship.
If a minor is 14 years of age or more he may select the person to whom he desires to be apprenticed.

DURATION OF APPRENTICESHIP—The duration of apprenticeship shall be in the case of the male until he arrives at the age of 21; and in the case of the female until she arrives at the age of 18 or until she marries in the event she marries before that age. (pp. 6–7)

In the 1921 version of *Texas Laws Made Plain,* the format and style, which included the question-and-answer format, posing questions like,"WHO SHOULD BE APPRENTICED," included more instances of active voice than Texas laws written during this same period. The 1921 plain language version is organized into more logical, numbered sections similar to the Plain English translations of apprenticeship laws in Appendix I of this book. Clearly, the plain language apprenticeship regulation published in the 1921 *Texas Laws Made Plain* manual was more accessible to those farmers with access to banks and written in a more user-friendly and clear format than the apprenticeship laws we discussed in Chapter 2 of this book. Unfortunately, we cannot herald the 1906 or 1921 *Texas Laws Made Plain* apprenticeship laws as a government-endorsed effort toward honesty or accessibility because, as I stated earlier in this chapter, apprenticeship regulations had been repealed since 1871. I searched the University of North Texas' full text online version of *Gammel's The Laws of Texas* (http://texinfo.library.unt.edu/lawsoftexas/search.htm), Volume 7 (1871) to Volume 20 (1921) and found no evidence of an apprenticeship law as outlined in the 1906 or 1921 version of the *Texas Laws Made Plain* manuals. In my online search, I did find brief references to specific counties having the authority to "apprenticeship minors as provided by law," but these references were mingled among lists of a host of other rights assigned to counties; in Texas law, there were no references to who might be apprenticed or the duration of apprenticeship as outlined in the manuals. It is significant that these short manuals of 100 pages, which according to the American National Bank in Austin, Texas provided plain language versions of "those provisions of the statutes believed to be of most concern to the people in general," does not include a reference to the year the laws were enacted nor a reference that would allow the reader to find the original versions of the laws (Simmons & Simmons, 1906, Preface). The 1906 and 1921 publications of Texas laws, for whatever reason, included a plain language version of an apprenticeship "law" that was not included in the 37th Texas Legislatures' publication of its 1921 Texas Laws or its supplement, nor was there a reference to a new apprenticeship law in the General Laws of Texas from 1920 to 1923. Thus, compliance with apprenticeship laws included in the plain language manuals meant that those who trusted the plain language version of the law had no way of knowing if the law was still enforceable or even in existence. Plain language apprentice laws written by the former attorney general of the state, like the Texas Black Codes, were inconsistent with laws of greater authority. The Texas Black Codes of 1866 were inconsistent with federal laws, and the plain language apprenticeship law in the *Texas Laws Made Plain* manuals published in 1906 and 1921 were inconsistent with Texas State laws.

While the writers of the Texas Black Codes intentionally left out words that would clearly address those black persons who would be the recipients of punishments and participants in unfair labor contracts, the Texas post-Reconstruction laws that followed were as harmful, but relied less on ambiguous text to support their enforcement. As years passed, post-Reconstruction laws redefined the word *apprentice* from the black child who was required to work for little or no money until age 21 to a person who was able to acquire a skill, join trade unions, and become self-employed. In 1947, after the establishment of the Texas State Board of Plumbing Examiners (Bureau of Labor Statistics, 1947, pp. 47–52), the term *apprentice* reappeared in labor-related Texas laws without any mention of the apprentice being bound or having to stay bound until the age of 21 or marriage:

> Chapter 115, Section 11. Apprentice
> Any person who has worked as a plumber's apprentice at the business, trade, or calling of plumbing for such a length of time as the Board may prescribe in its rules and regulations, and who desires to take an examination to entitle him to a license as a journeyman plumber, may file his application and take the examination provided by the Board. (Bureau of Labor Statistics, 1947, p. 52)

Years after the Freedman's Bureau's initial establishment of schools for children during Reconstruction, the State of Texas joined in this endeavor, establishing separate schools and colleges for black children to obtain education during the post-Reconstruction period. With the turn of the century, there was an obvious paradigm shift in the state's view of black children from laborers to students. Naturally, with this shift, came the deliberate effort by blacks to obtain certifications, licenses, and degrees that validated their skills and abilities, but there were still government-endorsed restrictions to labor for many black Texans. Like the Texas Black Codes, post-Reconstruction labor laws appeared to be "race neutral" because there was little or no reference to race nor was there any mention of the restrictions placed on blacks to practice trades. Surprisingly, there was no mention of race, even in those regulations that previously mentioned race (i.e., voting rights, civil responsibilities). In Section 295 of the Texas Labor Laws of 1923, blacks were not explicitly excluded from voting:

Section 295. Qualifications for voting: who not qualified.
The following classes of people shall not be qualified to vote in this state.
1. Persons under 21 years of age.
2. Idiots and lunatics.
3. All paupers supported by the county.
4. All persons convicted of any felony, except those restored to full citizenship and right of suffrage, or pardon.
5. All soldiers, marine or seaman, employed in the service of the array of army or navy of the United States. (Bureau of Labor Statistics, 1923, p. 177)

Despite the fact that Section 295 did not exclude blacks, and the Fifteenth Amendment of the United States Constitution guaranteed blacks the right to vote, voting was not without restrictions (i.e., poll tax and physical intimidation) for African Americans from post-Reconstruction until after the Voting Rights Act of 1964. Thus, like voting rights laws, the restrictions to the practice of trades by blacks in Texas were dependent on tacit laws, which were extensions of codified Texas law. Tacit law is "a law which derives its authority from the common consent of the people without any legislative enactment" (Black, 1990, p. 1452). Francis Bacon defined *tacit law* as "examples by which frequent use have passed into custom" (Bacon, 1858, p. 92). Those customs, exclusion of blacks from unions, supplemented legislative laws from post-Reconstruction to the Civil Rights Era and both worked together to create a formidable barrier that impeded the establishment of black labor in trade occupations that required licenses. According to Alwyn Barr,

> Black Texans in urban areas during the twentieth century found themselves limited primarily to unskilled jobs. As craft unions developed they literally closed printers, and miners. Tremendous urban demands for carpenters caused the number of black carpenters to double from 1900 to 1930 but combined with union exclusion to produce their decrease from 35 to 5 percent of all carpenters in the state." (Barr, 1996, p. 149)

Historically, union membership paved the career path from apprenticeship to journeymen to master tradespersons, and workers gained membership in unions through direct admissions and apprenticeships (University of Chicago Law Review, 1970, p. 343). Unwritten, yet understood, union laws and practices assured that black laborers would not gain entry through either path. In his 1936 article published in the *Journal of Negro Education*, A. Philip Randolph wrote, "Discrimination against the Negro workers by the trade union movement is doubtless the greatest challenge to its profession of democracy and its claim of representing progressive force in American Society (Randolph, 1936, p. 55). Although Randolph had been successful in organizing the Brotherhood of Sleeping Car Porters in 1936, when addressing unions in general, he stated,

> While inclusion of Negro workers in the trade union movement through the federal unions may be better than leaving them out entirely, the federal union is far from satisfactory, since Negro workers, in an industry which is covered by an agreement on wages and rules governing working conditions negotiated by an international union which excludes Negros, are impotent to change it, if perchance the agreement has provisions inimical to their interests. (p. 55)

Three years later and in the same journal, historian Charles H. Wesley's article, "The Present and Future Position of the Negro in the American Social Order," chronicled the effects of racial discrimination on trade union membership and the implications for black labor. Wesley described how white labor unions barred black participation directly through making union policies that excluded blacks or created separate unions for blacks and indirectly through examinations that tested applicants on algebra, physics, and trigonometry, coursework not directly related to the trades that used these examinations (University of Chicago Law Review, 1970, pp. 343–344; Wesley, 1939, p. 454). While most poorly educated blacks did not have the education to pass these tests, whites with similar levels of education could be admitted to unions through clauses that allowed admittance to family members and by obtaining letters of support from current white union members, letters that black laborers could not obtain (University of Chicago Law Review, 1970, p. 343). Thus, for decades, the Texas labor regulations ignored or endorsed discrimination in the labor and the practice of licensed trades, and these labor regulations were not useful to Texas blacks interested in gaining employment in the licensed trades these laws were supposed to make accessible.

RATIONALE FOR CONTEMPORARY STUDIES

The State of Texas' continued resistance to fair employment laws for blacks and other minorities is evident in the *State Fair Employment Laws and their Administration: Operations Manual Complementing the Civil Rights Act of 1964.* In 1964, when the book was published, Texas and other southern states did not have fair employment laws that made race-based discrimination "an unfair and unlawful employment practice for employers, labor unions, or employment agencies" (Bureau of National Affairs, 1964, p. 1).

During the years following desegregation and civil rights legislation, black laborers gained entry into industries and professions that had been long closed to them. While black employment in the trade and professional positions in the public and private sectors increased, some black small businesses that existed during segregation (i.e., black-owned movie theatres, grocery stores, and restaurants) closed as black consumers began to patronize white establishments. Although many black businesses closed after desegregation, black tradespersons requiring union membership and/or licenses, including plumbers, carpenters, beauticians, barbers, insurance agents, funeral home operators, elder-care facility operators, and daycare facility operators, gained prominence in black communities in Texas and throughout the nation. Today, these African American owned businesses are regulated entities, and the owners of these businesses are required to comply with Texas regulations and laws that have been rewritten to include them.

Barry Crouch explained that Texas Black Codes "maintained a nondiscriminatory facade that fooled no one" (1999, p. 264), and David Bernstein noted the continuation of this writing style throughout the southern States and argued, "facially neutral occupational regulations passed between the 1870s and the 1930s harmed African Americans. Sometimes racism motivated the laws, either directly (as when the sponsors of the legislation were themselves racists) or indirectly (when legislative sponsors responded to racism among their constituents" (2001, p. 5). Black Codes as well as labor regulations written during the first half of the 20th century used language to intentionally mask discrimination against blacks in regulations. The rhetorical analysis of the Texas Black Codes, *Texas Laws Made Plain,* and Texas laws from 1923 to 1947 grounded in the historical and cultural contexts in which these regulations were written support this argument.

In this chapter, I've attempted to provide the rationale for a contemporary study of black trust in the government with a focus on business regulations. In the results of a recent National Public Radio/Kaiser Family Foundation /Kennedy School study and poll, "Americans Distrust Government, but Want It to Do More," researchers found, "African Americans are much less likely to trust their state and local governments than whites are. Only about a quarter of African Americans say they trust their state government to do what is right just about always or most of the time; more than 40% of whites feel that way. Latinos are more likely to trust all levels of government" (National Public Radio, 2000, p. 1). Because African American distrust of government persists at a higher level than other populations, government agencies that are concerned with building trusting relationships with a distrustful African American population should certainly consider that a history of deceptively written and conflicting regulations contributes to African American trust in interactions with government agencies.

In the next chapter, I move my focus from the text of historical regulations to writers of contemporary regulations. I recount my interviews and observations of contemporary State of Texas regulatory writers and unveil the rhetorical strategies that they use to write regulations for historically distrustful audiences.

CHAPTER IV

Case Study II—
Texas Agencies:
The Challenge of Evoking Trust

In contemporary regulatory writing, preambles to regulations give the audience a glimpse of the contexts in which proposed and adopted regulations are invented, including public input. Still, the content of debates between the public and government personnel and debates within the government agency about word choice and style are often excluded from preambles; this information quickly fades into the collected memory of public policy writers, community activists, administrators, and attorneys. Contextual inquiry is a method that has proven successful in helping technical communicators identify tasks that writers and users perform in the production of texts as well as the tasks that audiences or users perform in understanding texts. "Contextual Inquiry gathers design data by sending individual designers to watch people do their job, interspersing observation, discussion, and reconstruction of past events" (Holtzblatt & Beyer, 1996, p. 308). In this chapter, I use contextual inquiry to excavate the writers' memories of the tasks they perform when writing regulations and unveil how they learn to write regulations and what types of information they privilege. Although government writing has been the focus of many publications in technical communication, few, if any, studies have been conducted to record the invention processes of regulatory writers or examine their attention to cultural factors, like race and trust. Dale Sullivan, a technical communication scholar, posits, "[if] we are serious about defining technical communication as a practice, then we must expand its scope to include political discourse" (1994, p. 228). To this end, the information analyzed in this portion of the study serves as a foundation to understanding how one type of political discourse, regulatory discourse, is written, as well as which voices are considered in the production of regulatory texts.

CONTEXTUAL INQUIRY MEETING AT STATE AGENCY

While the Texas Black Codes of 1866 are some of Texas' most deceptive regulations, and for blacks, early 20th-century labor regulations were voided by tacit laws, contemporary Texas agencies are attempting to write clear and honest regulations to help business owners of all ethnicities to understand and comply with the State of Texas. While the apprenticeship Texas Black Codes served to force black children to work and be punished as they had during slavery, the Texas Department of Family and Protective Services exists today to protect children of all ethnicities in daycares, family environments, and in living arrangements with adults outside of their family of origin. In November 1999, 133 years after the promulgation of Texas Black Codes and 78 years after the *Texas Laws Made Plain* latest edition referenced in this book, the Child Care Licensing Division of the Texas Department of Family and Protective Services announced its plan to review childcare licensing regulations by publishing a Notice of Intent in the *Texas Register*, the journal that publishes regulations and notices to solicit comments and suggestions from the public. After the Division received no opposition to this initiative, the agency made plans to rewrite regulations in Plain English. As suggested by scholars like Joseph Williams, the Child Care Licensing Division promptly began training attorneys, policy analysts, editors, and managers to "translate" regulations from legalese to Plain English (Williams, 1986, pp. 167–173).

Now, several years later, agency policy writers have rewritten hundreds of Child Care Licensing Division regulations in Plain English. In this chapter, I present a case study that focuses on responses collected in group meetings and individual interviews with three public-policy writers who, at the time of the meetings, were employed in the Child Care Licensing Division of the Texas Department of Family and Protective Services. Of the seven policy writers in this Division, three volunteered to participate in my study. These three subjects have experience writing regulations in legalese, Plain English, or both styles. The three volunteers were all female, and they were from ethnically diverse backgrounds. Since the childcare industry is predominately female, much of the inspection and regulation of this industry is also conducted by women.

Since contextual inquiry is a research method that allows the researcher to observe the subject in their work environment and ask questions about the tasks the subjects perform, I requested that participants allow me to observe them while writing regulations and interacting with attorneys, staff, and citizens. All participants agreed to be observed, until a week prior to my initial observation meeting, when I received an e-mail from one of the policy writers asking me if I really wanted to "observe" the writers or interview them and obtain an explanation of their rule writing process in a group setting. Basically, the e-mail informed me that a new set of regulations had just been submitted to the agency's Council for approval and few, if any, new regulations would be written until after the legislative session. The policy specialists would be busy responding to questions from legislators about the state of the agency, which at the time, was somewhat turbulent.

In the months prior to my contextual inquiry study, the agency's Child Protective Services Division had been under intense scrutiny from the media and the governor's office because of a number of child deaths that critics argued could have been prevented had the agency been more proactive in their investigations of child abuse. Although the Child Care Licensing Division, which is charged with enforcing regulations in childcare facilities, has different tasks than Child Protective Services, which handles child abuse and foster care facilities, the Texas Legislature's attention to the agency and its funding has affected the morale and outlook of the entire organization. With this in mind, I did not force the issue of spending 8 hours observing each policy writer and decided to allow the writers to show me as much of their environment as they were willing to share in their current political climate. Fortunately, the contextual inquiry method is designed to accommodate these changes; I was no longer going to spend several hours observing the policy writers write, but as you will see, I was eventually given entry into their environment, their writing processes, and their attitudes about their audiences.

On January 12, 2005, I began my contextual inquiry by meeting with policy writers in a room that they called the "crypt." In a group setting, which the policy writers seemed to prefer, I created a scenario that I hoped would reveal data pertinent to this study. Since I was no longer observing the policy writers write, I had to create an environment that would allow this information to surface without watching them sit in front of their computers and engage in the actual activity, while still being true to the contextual inquiry research method. In this effort, I attempted to simulate interaction between experienced policy writers and a novice by asking the policy writers how they would go about introducing a newly hired policy writer to regulatory writing in the Child Care Licensing Division. After a 2-hour discussion about what a new policy writer would need to know, including tasks and skills, I then met with each one individually in their cubicles, and they showed me the software and applications they used to write regulations, memos they created to communicate changes in policy, books they consulted, public comments, and regulation development flowcharts. Most importantly, they responded to several previously designed questions about their writing experiences, their perceptions of Plain English and legalese, and their consideration of historically marginalized audiences.

ARTIFACTS COLLECTED DURING CONTEXTUAL INQUIRY STUDY

Upon entry into the Child Care Licensing Division, the Associate Commissioner's administrative assistant greeted me, and she gave me copies of the volunteer and agency consent forms for my research. Soon after, Policy Writer B greeted me and informed me that she and the other policy writers would all meet me in the crypt momentarily; to keep the writers' responses confidential, I have given them the following pseudonyms: Policy Writer A, Policy Writer B, and Policy Writer C. Now, as a former project manager of rule development in this Division, I had spent many days in the crypt helping to plan statewide training sessions for Child Care Licensing enforcement staff and conducting rules meetings. The room had not changed much. The crypt is hidden in the back of the Division behind all of the Division offices and cubicles; it consists of a table and is surrounded by whiteboards, which were filled with texts about childcare regulations. Before the "meeting" began, Policy Writer B brought in a document that she stated would help me to understand the agency's new rule writing-processes. The document, titled "CCL Rules Process" includes 32 steps, starting with the subject-matter expert preparing a draft and ending with implementation of the policy. The document, which contains names of personnel at the agency, is not included in this book, but each step in the document is analyzed later in this chapter.

Later, while speaking with Policy Writer A in her cubicle, I was given another document, titled "Cross-Agency Rulemaking Process Consolidation Project: Proposed Rulemaking Process for DFSP, DARS, DADS, & DSHS." This document included a 52-step flowchart created to help the policy writers understand the new regulation approval processes as a draft moves from the policy writer to publication in the *Texas Register*. I made note of style- and invention-related references in all of these documents in the discourse analysis of data gathered in the contextual inquiry portion of this chapter.

PROCESS MEETING WITH GROUP OF POLICY WRITERS

Once the three policy writers arrived in the crypt, I began the meeting with a description of my research and described the contextual inquiry data-collection method. I informed the writers that contextual inquiry allows the researcher to go into a workplace, observe the work environment, tasks, and ask questions about various processes. I stated that the method was very flexible, which is suitable for meetings like this one, where I'll simply ask them to describe a process and clarify information as we progressed. Finally, I stated, "I'd like for you to explain the rule writing process at Child Care Licensing. Please explain it to me as if I was a new employee with policy writing responsibilities." I asked, "What tools will I need? Who will I need to talk to? What style of writing should I use? What type of training will I need?" I asked the policy writers to focus on the writing process as opposed to the content of the regulations. I attempted to document the policy writers' responses verbatim, but I have paraphrased some responses for clarity. The fact that I had previously worked with two of the policy writers and shared much of their knowledge about rule writing may explain why their responses were somewhat technical and void of definitions and clarifications. Basically, the policy writers went directly into an in-depth conversation about why they write, how they write, and a description of stakeholders who inform their revision process.

Clearly, the policy writers who volunteered to participate in my study are more ethnically diverse and are of a different gender than those legislators who wrote Texas Black Codes, and they certainly operate in a very different political and social environment than did the postbellum Texas Black Codes. It is also clear that the content of the regulations are much different than the Texas Black Codes. Still, it seems that contemporary policy writers still struggle with finding a balance between communicating the agency's intent to protect their own interests as well as the interests of the reader.

ANALYSIS OF REGULATORY WRITING TASKS

Thomas Barker describes tasks as "well-defined effort[s] of short duration" and argues, "because of their well-defined nature, tasks are independent of one another" (1998, p. 99) Although the Child Care Licensing (CCL) Rule Process flowchart includes 52 steps, these steps actually fall under six independent tasks—writing the rule, notifying internal and external stakeholders of the policy change, editing the rule, receiving feedback from those decision makers and stakeholders, approving the rule, and adopting and implementing the rule. In this chapter, I discuss the information in the CCL Rules Process flowchart as well as information collected during my interviews and observations of the policy writers. Their voices are used to construct a narrative of rule writing from the writers' perspective, not from the agency executives who approved the CCL Rules Process flowchart but from those persons who actually write the regulations.

The first major task that emerged in my content analysis of the CCL Rules Process flowchart was the actual drafting of the rules. In Figure 4.1, the information listed under the "Write" category suggests that all of the drafting or incorporating of changes is done by one group, the "SMEs" or subject-matter experts. The subject-matter experts write the initial draft of the rule, incorporate changes suggested by reviewers, and incorporate public comments and responses to public comments in the preamble of rules. Although rule writing is a collaborative writing process, it is clear that the responsibility of revising the

54 / FROM BLACK CODES TO RECODIFICATION

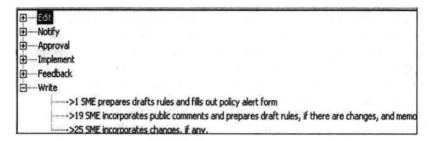

Figure 4.1. Writing regulations.

draft to make sure that all voices are included in the final draft of the proposed and adopted rules is the responsibility of the Child Care Licensing subject-matter experts, also called policy writers.

In this chapter, I discuss specific information about rule writing, including rule writing tasks, that the group of Child Care Licensing policy writers provided in both their individual and group interviews. Although I did not explicitly pose these questions to the policy writers, their responses could be used to answer the following questions:

1. What information is contained in rules?
2. What actions initiate rule writing activities?
3. What research is required to write a rule?
4. How does a writer promote consistency in rules?
5. Who reviews and approves rules?
6. What happens when personnel changes occur?
7. How do policy writers learn to write rules?
8. Who owns the rules?

According to the policy writers, a new policy writer would need to be introduced to this information to understand the tasks associated with rulemaking. The second set of information that I'll use to give voice to those who actually write the regulations is the information collected from the individual meetings with Child Care Licensing policy writers when policy writers discussed their individual writing processes.

In these discussions, the writers revealed their expertise in the rule writing as well as some areas where they lacked knowledge concerning the needs of their agency and audience. Now that I've identified the themes that emerged from my interaction with the policy writers, it is important that we take a look at what the policy writers wanted to tell the fictional new policy writer about writing rules.

In the group meeting with the simulated training session with Child Care Licensing policy writers, the participants thought it important to define "rule" for the new policy writer or answer the question, "What is rule?" Statements such as, "We make sure that Policy Clarifications are in rule. How-to-complys must be in rule," suggests that in the past, the agency has had several types of policy that they used to regulate child care facilities—rules, standards, and policy clarification memos. Phrases like, "We are much clearer now about how rules are different from policies and procedures" and "We can't put things in policy without it being in rule" hint that there had been some confusion within the agency regarding what information should be adopted as rule and what information should be included in the Minimum Standards, which are the policies Child Care Licensing inspectors had previously used to cite violations of agency requirements. Hypothetically, after a childcare licensing representative inspected a facility, the inspector could have had the authority to cite state law, rule, or minimum standards, which were referenced in state law. The writers posited that they needed to propose and adopt requirements in policy clarification memos as well as minimum standards into rule to make all of the policy consistent and enforceable. Basically, the policy writers presented arguments for the same language in rules and handbooks—they wanted consistent and memorable information for both regulation enforcers and regulated entities. Policy writers thought it important that they communicate to the "new policy writer" not only what a rule was but also what actions initiate rule writing activities. The writers identified the sources of rule writing activities—internal and external to the government agency. They also communicated the types of issues that would serve as impetuses for proposed new rules, including calls from legislators and recurring problems mentioned by government agency field staff or inspectors and childcare providers.

Donald Murray argued, "Prewriting is everything that takes place before the first draft. Prewriting usually takes about 85% of the writer's time. . . . Prewriting may include research and daydreaming, notemaking and outlining, title-writing and lead-writing" (1997, p. 4). In their discussions of their individual writing process, like Murray, the policy writers also counted thinking and note taking as an important part of their writing process. One writer explained, "I start by thinking about our mission," "I think about the internal stakeholders," "I have an idea about what I want to say, what is important," "What are the important elements that I want to cover." Even after thinking about the mission and audience, the writers mention several other tasks before starting a draft on their computers. Writers mention sharing notes from meetings to make sure that they understand discussions about policy, clarifying definitions in meetings with agency staff and attorneys before retreating to their computers and using Microsoft Word to write an initial draft.

Karen Burke LeFevre argues, "many of us have indeed read 'autonomous themes' (and perhaps written them ourselves in English 101) in which the writer and the writing seem asocial, and invention appears to occur in a vacuum," but she goes on to argue that no invention is asocial (1987, p. 17). The same can be said of the invention of regulatory discourse. The policy writers were forthright about the assistance from peers and attorneys in constructing preliminary drafts of regulations. Their remarks suggest that the collaborative writing aspect of rule invention is the main source of training for new policy writers. Writers stated they learned how to write policies by, "working in teams and asking questions," "by just doing it," "you learn by examples from your coworkers, working together as a group," and "we have to work with the automation staff to see how the regulation change will affect Class, the automation system for our division."

In addition to collaboration within the agency, policy writers also resort to external resources and conduct research when making initial drafts of regulations. In the policy writers' discussions of research they conduct when writing rules, they mentioned consulting national organizations that have general standards regarding "what good out-of-home care is." In *Lesson-Drawing in Public Policy* by Richard Rose, this type of policy analysis is called "Lesson Drawing." Rose argues,

> In the policy process a lesson can be defined as a program for action based on a program or programs undertaken in another city, state, or nation by the same organization in its own past. Lessons can be drawn across time, as in frequently invoked "lessons in history." An organization's own past is one fruitful source of experience, but lessons can also be drawn across space. (1993, p. 21)

The policy writers also mentioned that they also use this same maneuver in their writing processes; the writers look at other states who use the Plain English question-and-answer format as a reference when writing in Plain English.

In the individual meetings with the policy writers, the writers continued their discussions of lesson drawing from other states. Two writers mentioned that they used the Internet as well as in-office references to find information about how other states write rules and the content of those rules. At the time of this study, e-rulemaking activities were not a part of this agency's rule writing processes. One writer's mention of the use of Microsoft Excel as a research tool was not clear until I observed copies of a variety of spreadsheets created using Microsoft Excel and saved for future reference. Each policy writer's personal workspace included a cubicle space, a white board, personal computer, table and chairs for collaboration and guests, and a window view. Although the work environments for each policy writer were very similar, the reference documents saved on their hard drives were vastly different. As I observed the policy writer's work environments, the workers showed me diverse research-related materials that they created, updated, and referenced when writing rules. It was obvious that many of the internal documents that policy writers reference are created for their own personal use, but what happens to these documents if they move to another agency or position?

Tacit knowledge is "our ability to recognize faces without knowing how we do so, and to be trained in a psychological laboratory to respond to certain perceived stimuli without knowing just what it is we are responding to" (Bothamely, 2002, p. 518). In their attempts to explain how they wrote regulations, the policy writers referred to themselves as "gatekeepers" and "subject-matter experts" without any clear explanation of how they obtained their expertise, knowledge, or training. The policy writers mention the fact that "knowledge bases," a term they understood and embraced when I used it, are often lost when staff change, but they could not explain how knowledge was obtained.

Policy writers use internal reference materials to write regulations; these resources serve as tools that facilitate the policy writers' training. For example, the Microsoft Excel spreadsheet that one policy writer used to keep record of over 16,000 public comments that the agency received in response to the Plain English translation and revision of the Child Care Licensing daycare regulations contains a wealth of knowledge regarding public opinion about the Division's rules. At the time of the interview, the enormous size of the file the document was stored in made it inaccessible to other policy writers. The creator of the document stated that she understood that it would probably better serve the whole agency if it were placed on the network drive, but it would probably take up too much space. Other documents that the writers kept on their hard drives were derivation tables. One writer explained, "We use derivation tables, which we create in Microsoft Excel, to keep track of rule changes. These tables tell us where rules originate, why we create a rule, the difference between old and new rules and standards, and puts old and new language back to back. We can see how the rule has changed by looking at the table."

Despite the research that the writers perform and collect, the writers explained the difficulties they encounter when presenting research to support "leaving the rules as they are." One writer suggested that policy writers use their research to argue the status quo, but it is often difficult to persuade new administrators or agency executives that rules should not be changed. The comments reflect the fact that policy writers feel the need to defend the rules to each new administrator.

The second major task that emerged from the Child Care Licensing process flowchart concerned the "notify" category. The agency's Rule Coordinator, who serves as the project manager for the agency's rule development process, spends quite a bit of time making sure that other agencies, internal agency staff charged with implementing regulations, and the public, are notified of the Child Care Licensing division's intent to change rules. The Division is required by law to publish proposed rule changes in the *Texas Register* for public comment, but notification of field staff and internal staff is just as important; the rule writers must obtain buy-in and support from internal as well as external stakeholders to make rule changes.

In Lisa Ede and Andrea Lunsford's seminal article, "Audience Addressed/ Audience Invoked: The Role of Audience in Composition Theory and Pedagogy," the authors posit, "Those who envision audience as addressed emphasize the concrete reality of the writer's audience; they also share the assumption that knowledge of the audience's attitude, beliefs, and expectations is not only possible (via observation and analysis) but essential" (1997, p. 78). The policy writers were quick to refer me to the agency's real audience, that audience revealed in the 52-step process that highlights a specific audience, which includes people identified through their positions inside and outside of the Child Care Licensing Division. Most of this audience or those persons required to read (review) all proposed rules before adoption by the agency are real, and the policy writers can meet them and negotiate the language and intent of the proposed rules. At the time of the contextual inquiry meetings, the Child Care Licensing Division had recently changed their governing body from a board of directors to a council, which the writers state has less power than the former board structure. These internal stakeholders are ultimately responsible for the promulgation of all rules and thus, have a great deal of responsibility for making certain that rules are effective in protecting children. Another body that oversees the internal activities of the Child Care Licensing Division is the Texas Health and Human Services Commission, which is charged with approving and overseeing the activities of all Texas state agencies that provide and enforce Health and Human Services regulations. The main issue that the policy writers mentioned in relation to this audience, which they address, was how much or how little power the different audiences have when reviewing their rules. The writers were concerned with how many internal stakeholders have to review their regulations, as well as whether the input or opinions of these stakeholders will affect the final language of their proposed regulation.

Policy writers mentioned several methods that they used to involve external stakeholders, such as advocacy groups, nonprofit organizations, and the regulated entities. Clearly, these groups fall outside of the agency, and their interests range from the health and safety of the children to financial gain. The policy writers stated that they use workgroups and focus groups to inform and obtain feedback from the external stakeholders. Interestingly enough, the notification of external stakeholders in groups is not included in the Division's 52-step rule development process. Both focus groups and workgroups are reserved for those special occasions when the policy writer is attempting to obtain buy-in or feedback from external stakeholders, but the policy writers have flexibility because the law does not require that the agency hold focus groups or workgroup meetings for every proposed rule. If this type of external input were required, the rule writing and development process would be longer and more expensive.

Despite the fact that most of the subject positions mentioned in the 52-step review process can be linked to people that the policy writers can speak with and know, there is one important segment of the audience involved in the review process that the writers cannot know personally but should certainly analyze; this audience is called "the public." In the Division's 52-step rule development process, the public is formally involved when the proposed regulation is published in the *Texas Register* for "public comment." When I asked the policy writers about the demographic makeup of this public audience, their responses were not nearly as clear as the description of the internal audience laid out in the process chart. The writers described the ethnicity of their audience as "reflective of Texas," "The ethnicity is probably similar to the national average," and "mostly white . . . maybe?" One policy writer was less vague and stated, "I write regulations for criminal background checks of providers, and this disproportionately affects minorities." Because of Texas' growing Latino population, we can assume that the minorities served by this agency include African Americans, Hispanics, and in some parts of Texas, a growing Asian population. While one policy writer expressed concern regarding difficulties in communicating with the growing Vietnamese-speaking population in Houston and Arlington, Texas, another admitted, "The system is lacking because we don't consider that minority families have different family practices. . . . There is distrust among providers."

A government agency or "system" that acknowledged practices and values would be attempting to demonstrate cultural competence. Layla P. Suleiman argues that issues related to cultural competence in communicating with Latinos with limited English proficiency (LEP) is more than a communication issue, but it is quite possibly a legal issue that results in civil rights violations (2003, p. 185). With the growing Latino population in the United States, Suleiman posits an increasing need for government agencies, particularly social services agencies, to provide bilingual services and "written policies" about language accessibility for people with limited language proficiency (p. 190). She links demographics revealing a growing Latino population and excerpts from the following civil rights legislation to argue that cultural competency, as it relates to communication with Latinos with LEP, is a legal requirement: "no person in the United States shall on the ground of race, color or national origin, be excluded from participation in, be denied the benefits of, or be subjected to discrimination under any program or activity receiving Federal financial assistance" (Suleiman, 2003, p. 190).

Suleiman provides poignant examples of how some government agencies' refusal to provide services that were needed in order to be culturally competent (i.e., reluctance to hire bilingual staff or reluctance to train staff about cultural differences) can lead to violations of the law (p. 189). For example, Suleiman provides an example that describes how in some cases, Latino children who speak

English may be asked to translate for their LEP parents when communicating with child abuse investigators, even in cases where the LEP parent is the suspected abuser. Another example includes the frequent request for neighbors or associates to translate for LEP individuals requesting services from the government; in these cases, Suleiman suggests that there is no way of discerning whether the translators, who gain no tangible benefit from being honest arbitrators, are intentionally misrepresenting information, to the detriment of the LEP client (p. 194).

Suleiman presents a variety of perspectives related to cultural competence, but there is very little guidance about how this concept, though clearly defined, is measured. She suggests that cultural competence as it relates to language access for Latinos with limited English proficiency should not only be a standard, but incorporated in written policies (p. 190). On the surface, this might seem fair and even practical, but the implementation of cultural competence as a standard or law is actually very complex. The complexity of such criteria is based on the fact that such standards must have clear and measurable goals to determine whether or not they can be reached. What criteria should organizations use to determine whether an individual is culturally competent? If a criterion for meeting cultural competence in government organizations when serving Latino populations means that the government employee is fluent in Spanish, similar efforts toward cultural competence, as outlined in the last chapter of this book, can be used for those government employees communicating with populations where citizens are distrustful of government agencies.

In my contextual inquiry study, one policy writer suggested that regardless of the ethnic background of the audience, "The main thing is that the rules are clear and of the best interests of the children." This same policy writer stated, "We need to consider the children and their voice." These statements are important because they describe how regulatory writing can differ from many other types of technical communication, where the technical communicator serves as an advocate for the user. In regulatory writing, the user or reader is often not the first person that the policy writer/technical communicator is concerned with; these writers are writing on behalf of the children. So, in addition to the writer, audience, and text, the regulatory writer invokes this public audience by using the agency's voice as well as the voice of its constituent. Does the fact that the writer is not as much an advocate for the reader as for the children set regulatory writing apart from other types of technical writing? Does the fact that the writer has to incorporate these two voices—the agency's organizational voice as well as the children's voice—make the job of audience analysis and evoking trust in certain audience less probable or even less important? Ede and Lunsford posit,

> Those who envision audience as invoked stress that the audience of a written discourse is a construction of the writer. . . . The central task of the writer, then, is not to analyze an audience and adopt discourse to meet

its needs. Rather, the writer uses the semantic and syntactic resources of language to provide cues for the reader—cues which help to define the role or roles the writer wishes the reader to adopt in responding to the text. (1997, pp. 82–83)

Thus, if the policy writer is demanding that the reader meet certain minimum standards in childcare, it may not matter what ethnicity the audience is; but the writer should cue the audience so that they can adapt to the role of proficient childcare provider. In regulatory discourse, these textual cues can certainly be effective if the regulatory agency has encouraged the public to help negotiate the language, tone, and content of the regulation through feedback.

In rule writing, feedback is the impetus for revision. The third major task that emerged from the Child Care Licensing process flowchart also concerned the "notify" category. The writers described situations where the agency's policy writers solicited and received feedback from internal and external stakeholders. Most of this feedback was related to the content, not the style of the rule. The writer's opportunity to consider both the content and style of rules occurred during the fourth major task found in the Child Care Licensing process flowchart, the "edit" category. The editing stage included the routing and editing tasks that involve the agency editor, project manager, and staff responsible for formatting and editing the rules for publication in the *Texas Register* and preparing the rules package for the Council meeting. The *Texas Register,* like the *Federal Register,* has specific style guides that regulatory writers and editors must follow before rules are published for public review. The *Texas Register Format and Style Guide* speaks less to the style of the rule than to the arrangement of the rule and its preamble. Thus, the rules editor is responsible for making certain that the preamble contains all expected parts and that the rule's subsections are formatted correctly. The rules editor is also responsible for making certain that the rules are correct in punctuation and grammar.

Stella Ting-Toomey posits, "To develop trust, we have to understand the cultural meanings behind the words 'trust' and 'trustworthiness.' Trust means to rely on the consistency of someone's credibility, words, behaviors, actions, or network support. Trustworthiness means to make our own behaviors or actions worthy of the trust of others" (1999, p. 223). In *A Plain English Handbook: How to Create Clear SEC Documents,* the authors suggest that "reading the same material two or three times can bore and even trouble readers" (Securities and Exchange Commission, 1998, p. 12). Child Care Licensing policy writers confirm that they are attempting to be consistent across agency documents and reduce redundancy. One policy writer stated, "The benefits of consolidating standards is consistency; when you have too many sets of standards it's difficult." To this end, the policy writers are not only attempting to increase consistency but to decrease duplication or redundant regulations that increase the possibility of inconsistent enforcement of regulations.

In the Child Care Licensing Division, policy writers responses to my questions about the Plain English and legalese styles of writing suggests neither style is more appropriate. They stated, "We found out a year after the Plain English minimum standards were adopted that the rules still need to be clarified," "We found out the hard way that Plain English doesn't negate the need for more training," "The need to clarify and the inability for field staff to make judgments is still a problem in Plain English," "No matter what kind of rule you write, there are always all types of problems that pop up that you don't expect," "legalese left more room for field staff and providers to be subjective," "providers used legalese against the agency because of the wiggle room," and "they can't have it both ways, clarity and objectivity." Many of these arguments by policy writers who were not attorneys, sound eerily similar to arguments that attorney's use to justify legalese. Hilary Frooman posits that lawyers are taught that some legal terms are only definable in context and so their writing avoids defining "terms of art" or legal terms like "contract," because defining these words could compromise their legal positions (1981, p. 46). Frooman argues, "Lawyers will not accept plain English gratefully or willingly. Because an attorney can never predict how a judge will decide a case, or what argument his opponent will use, he is often reluctant to make strong statements" (p. 50). Thus, lawyers are following Aristotle's advice in that "If, then, the action is indefinable when a law must be framed, it is necessary to speak in general terms, so that if someone wearing a ring raises his hand or strikes, by the written law is violating the law and does wrong, when in truth he has [perhaps] not done any harms, and this [after judgment] is fair" (1991, p. 105). In this book, the question is not whether the language in laws and regulations leaves room for interpretation given unexpected circumstances, but whether laws and regulations are phrased in a language and form that is so obscure that it evokes distrust in its audience.

If we evaluate policy writer responses about style, we would be forced to concede, as have the writers, that both the Plain English and legalese styles are difficult to understand, fail to respond to unexpected circumstances that regulatory bodies must respond to, and will never be subjective enough for some or objective enough for others. With this said, there are still areas where editing and revision can help, and those are certainly related to areas of trust. Trust is the issue involved when the *ethos* of the agency might lead the audience or reader to react in one of two ways when regulations are not as clear as that particular reader would like: (1) the audience might telephone, write, or e-mail the agency for clarification or (2) the audience might place the regulation aside and hope that their business is somehow compliant. Every government agency in this country has an obligation to its citizenry to prefer the first. Most, if not all government agencies in this country are provided the means, not only to regulate, but also to explain its regulations. Thus, if the regulation promotes trust, it might also promote dialogue.

In my professional experience working in regulatory agencies, I observed policy writers who had written in legalese for years and were certainly not welcoming to the Plain English style of writing, just as many people who are computer illiterate have an unhealthy aversion to information technology. The policy writers in this study did not express any strong inclination or writing experience in either Plain English or legalese. In this study, the policy writers stated that they either did not have any prior experience writing in legalese or had some experience writing in Plain English and legalese. None of the policy writers had written in legalese more than 2 years before starting to translate regulations from legalese to Plain English. As it relates to regulatory writing, the participants in this study are relatively new to this genre of technical communication.

The Child Care Licensing policy writers discussed legalese from two perspectives: how they felt about writing in that style and their audience's perceptions of the style. The policy writers were careful to state the pros and cons that they accorded this style and made no blanket condemnation of it. One writer thought that the benefits of legalese included the fact that it supports their need to not "box ourselves in" and their need for "flexibility to use judgment." Another stated that legalese is "easier to write." On the other hand, the writers suggested that their audience does not "understand legalese or apply it." Another writer stated that the legalese style "requires more thought," and "has too much wiggle room." The writers' perception of the Plain English style, was often expressed in terms of regret or disappointment. It's clear that the Plain English style has not afforded the writers the benefits that they expected. Statements such as, "I thought Plain English would be easier, but I still get questions from field staff about what things mean," "We have to do a lot of interpreting with Plain English," "The number of rules increase as we translate them," "It's hard to write something that is clear and not too prescriptive," and several other statements about this style suggests that it is not as effective as the writers expected. After reflecting on the challenges associated with the Plain English style, it was still apparent that the policy writers agreed with the one policy writer who stated that she believed Plain English was more effective. In looking at the contexts in which the writer made this claim, I realized that this writer meant in terms of how much more thought was required of the reader in order to understand the legalese texts. In her complete statement, the subject said, "I believe Plain English is more effective. Legalese requires more thought. There is consideration of a new 'Rationale' document that providers can use that includes the rationale or interpretation of the regulation." Thus, although the regulations have been translated into Plain English, the writer feels that the Plain English style, though it sometimes lacks an adequate rationale or interpretation of the regulation, at the very least it requires the reader to think less. Certainly, proponents of Lacan and others might argue that regulations that require the audience to engage in less thought are too simplistic (Lather, 1996, p. 528), but those of us who acknowledge that the goal of childcare regulations is to promote health and safety and not the creation of new meaning can, therefore, understand this policy writer's argument. To support this argument, the policy writer who stated that legalese was easier to write, stated that "Plain English is more difficult to write" and "Plain English makes the writers ask themselves what they really mean." This is a powerful statement in that it suggests that legalese with all of its clauses and dense texts allows the writer to write without fulfilling their purpose, which is to communicate the subject matter. So, although the reader may be doing less thinking when reading Plain English regulations, the writer is not.

The fifth major task that emerged from the Child Care Licensing process flowchart was in the "approval" category. In the approval stage, other genres of technical communication are also routed for approval. The rule is accompanied by a fiscal impact form, which the project manager uses to collect information for the rule preamble and a Council memorandum, which the project manager uses to persuade the agency Council of the exigency for the proposed rule change. If these documents are approved and signed by agency decision makers, the rules are approved by agency staff, adopted, and published to notify the public. Then, agency staff are trained for implementation of new rules. Of course, there are numerous steps required to implement the regulation, including updating Web sites, internal handbooks, brochures, and forms that are not included as part of the rule development process. Still, the updating of these technical documents is crucial to the effective implementation of rules.

Another important issue the policy writers wanted to communicate to a fictional "new policy writer" was the collaborative nature of regulatory writing. One subject stated, "I understand the public process, but it's painful to see the rule changes." Another stated, "We will totally lose ownership once the legislators review rules." These statements suggest that subject-matter experts and rule writers must be prepared for numerous changes to their initial drafts, including the disregard of information that the writers perceive as important. This is the nature of regulatory writing and, oftentimes, collaborative writing in general.

Finally, it was obvious that the Child Care Licensing policy writers considered their translation of regulations from legalese to Plain English an accomplishment. The policy writers suggested that other agencies were "looking for copies of our daycare standards." They also asserted that "We are Texas," which gave them the license to be innovative and try new initiatives in their regulatory writing style. There may be some truth to this argument, which sounded a lot like the slogans "Texas, It's Like A Whole Other Country"™ or "Don't Mess with Texas,"™ which state agencies use to promote Texas pride and borders on braggadocio. While Texas has a history of sending plain-spoken yet charismatic politicians to national and state office, including Presidents Lyndon B. Johnson and George W. Bush and Governor Ann Richards, acceptance of plain-spoken politicians in Texas might have actually been set by Texas's first female governor, Miriam "Ma" Ferguson, who ran for governor in 1924 after her husband, Governor James Ferguson, was impeached. Ferguson was elected governor of Texas despite her campaign against the Ku Klux Klan and after running under the campaign slogan "Two governors for the price of one" (Huddleston, 2001, p. 1). This history of plain-spoken politicians and acceptance of the "plain-folks appeal" in political campaigns signals an acceptance of this general style of communication in interactions between the Texas public and its government (Lowenstein, 1981, p. 89). In the next chapter, I'll present user-centered data that evaluates a particular audience's perception of contemporary Texas regulations; we'll see if an audience of African American business owners in Austin, Texas view Plain English regulations as clear, innovative, and most importantly for this study, trustworthy.

CHAPTER V

Case Study III—
Contemporary Black Business Owners: Legalese, Plain English, or Both?

While conducting my research on contemporary regulatory writing and the responses of black business owners in Austin, Texas, I could not ignore the circumstances surrounding the destruction of two prominent African American-owned businesses in this city. I'd be remiss not to mention the accidental burnings of these two black-owned businesses or in failing to compare the divergent responses to these tragedies from local government officials. In October 2004, the loss of Dot's Restaurant, a local soul food restaurant frequented by Austinites of all ethnicities and cultures and owned by an elderly African American woman, resulted in an outpouring of financial and emotional support from the Austin community. In the days following the accident, thousands of people, including the Austin city mayor, visited the site of Dot's and left condolences as well as contributions for the rebuilding of this Austin landmark.

Approximately 4 months later, Austin, the self-proclaimed "Live Music Capitol of the World," suffered the loss of the African American community's most popular R&B club, Midtown Live, which was mostly frequented by African Americans in the Austin community. As Midtown Live burned and the local news correspondents and camera people surrounded the club to get video footage for the morning news, an African American woman, who looked on as the club burned, happened to peer through an Austin police officer's patrol car and noticed that the following phrase appeared on the police officer's computer interface: "Burn, Baby Burn." The woman did well to quickly show the computer interface and the now infamous phrase to camerapersons from local news stations that videotaped it for all to see. This night was followed by weeks of dialogue, controversy, and apologies about the phrase that the woman just so happened to see. After a quick and thorough internal investigation of the events of that night,

City of Austin officials revealed that not one but several Austin police officers had sent text messages over police communication technologies that expressed a lack of sympathy and sensitivity for the owners of the club, whose establishment burned as they watched. While one officer wrote, "U can smell from [Interstate] 35. It is the smell of victory"; a dispatcher wrote, "I have some extra gasoline if they need it," ("Texas Cops," 2005). Clearly, the city officials and police officers had drastically different experiences regulating the activities of the quaint soul food restaurant and a busy night club that reportedly kept police officers busy with over one hundred complaints in 2003 ("Texas Cops," 2005). Still, I tell these two stories, one of an outpouring of care for the loss of a business that the Austin community-at-large enjoyed and another of the "concealed" celebration of the ruin of a black-owned business that almost exclusively benefited the black community, to highlight reasons why many African American business owners continue to mistrust the stewards of the public trust.

In April 2006, the Minority Business Development Agency (MBDA), the U.S. Census, and the National Black Chamber of Commerce announced a 45% increase in the number of African American-owned businesses between 1997 and 2002 to 1.2 million. African American-owned businesses generate almost $89 billion in revenues and employ over 750,000 people (U.S. Department of Commerce, 2006). Although the increase in the number of businesses is remarkable, the revenues generated are discernibly less than any of the top 10 Fortune 500 companies in 2006 (CNN.com, 2006). Still, the rapid growth in the number of black-owned businesses is a sign that African Americans are indeed interested in creating wealth and jobs through entrepreneurship. So, in the midst of this growth, I examine the perceptions of government regulations by African American business owners in Texas. Specifically, in this chapter, I present voices representing Austin business owners and their responses to contemporary regulatory writing. Although my focus group meeting with some of these business owners was held a few weeks prior to the "Burn, Baby Burn" incident, you would not necessarily know that from some of the responses of some of the focus group members. The focus group participants were, without doubt, distrustful of government regulators. This chapter will explore African American distrust to see if it extends beyond government agencies and personnel to the invention and style of government regulations.

Six African American business owners were selected to participate in this focus group study, including one married couple. All focus group participants own businesses located within 50 miles of Austin. The sources used to obtain the subjects include the *Black Registry,* which is a local publication listing many Austin-area businesses owned by blacks; the *Black Registry* is published by a local African American-owned newspaper, the *Villager.* Other subjects were solicited through the Capital City African-American Chamber of Commerce newsletter and through personal and business contacts. All volunteers were recruited using a recruitment letter, which was included in an issue of the Capital

City African-American Chamber of Commerce Newsletter and mailed or e-mailed directly to African American business owners. Also, business owners were contacted via telephone and/or e-mail to follow up on the initial recruitment effort. The focus group was conducted in a meeting room at the Austin History Center, located next to the main branch of the Austin Public Library.

Approximately 2 weeks before the focus group meeting, all volunteers were provided a brief overview of the study using a recruitment letter and asked to study four examples of contemporary regulations written in Plain English and legalese and respond to a pre-focus group questionnaire about the effectiveness of the styles of regulatory writing. While the focus group participants stated that they reviewed the regulations in the questionnaire, only three subjects submitted the questionnaire. Prior to the focus group meeting, I used the completed questionnaire responses to help shape the focus group questions. By coupling the questionnaire with the focus group questions, I attempted to duplicate the procedure in "Revising Safety Instructions with Focus Groups" by Rien Elling (1997). In his study, Elling wrote, "A couple of days before the session [focus group], the participants reviewed the text with the request to mark the text with plus and minus signs while reading it: a plus sign if they agreed with the text or found the information important, useful clear, readable, exactly what they wanted to know, easy to apply practice oriented, and so on and a minus sign where they had the opposite opinion" (p. 457). Although I did not use the plus and minus signs, I did ask each subject to review the two styles, Plain English and legalese, of Child Care Licensing regulations and prompted them with questions that I hoped would solicit responses that highlighted text that the subjects viewed as negative or positive and evoked trust or distrust. In the focus group meeting, the subjects were given additional time to review the same regulations included on the pre-focus group meeting questionnaire (two of the regulations were written in Plain English and two in legalese) before being prompted for their responses to the regulations.

To facilitate the meeting, I solicited the help of a professional counselor, Thereisa Coleman, who has experience conducting group-counseling sessions. My role in the meeting was to document subject responses using only my laptop computer and to ask for clarifications and additional responses when necessary. The pre-focus group questionnaire, participant responses, focus group questions, and focus group responses are documented in the following section. Again, I used pseudonyms to protect the identity and confidentiality of the subjects. Subject A is the owner of a food establishment, Subject B owns a financial services company, Subject C owns a retail establishment, Subjects D and E are co-owners of two health care facilities, and Subject F owns a building maintenance company. The regulations these subjects reviewed are current Plain English and recently repealed legalese regulations promulgated by the Child Care Licensing Division of the Texas Department of Family and Protective Services, the same division that I observed in the contextual inquiry portion of this book. I purposely avoided recruiting childcare facility owners because in a similar pilot study, I found that subjects are less likely to criticize regulations they are required to follow, possibly out of fear of personal, negative repercussions. The results of my pilot study suggest that in studies assessing audience perceptions of Plain English and legalese regulations, researchers should include an "outsider" or participant who is not a government employee, paid consultant, or entity regulated by the texts under scrutiny. By including the outsider, who is not afraid of the regulatory agency and is not an employee of the agency and endorsing most of its proposals, the researcher can obtain new and objective data about preferred styles of regulatory writing from energetic and critical participants. The subjects in this study were certainly energetic, critical, and most were active participants in the focus group meeting. While one participant described the meeting as therapeutic and stated that he needed to discuss these issues with other African American business owners more often, another stated that at his age he had nothing to hide and would willingly forfeit any confidentiality to voice his opinions about this subject.

I began the focus group by introducing the facilitator and myself and thanking the subjects for participating in the study. I briefly described my research objectives and explained that I would be taking notes while the facilitator asked questions that I had prepared prior to the meeting. I assured the participants that the focus group meeting would not exceed the agreed upon timeframe, 1 hour, and reminded them that the information collected would be confidential. The facilitator then began the meeting by passing out a 2-page document, which included the contemporary regulations from the pre-focus group questionnaire that were written in legalese and Plain English. The actual transcript of the focus group meeting, including the questions posed by the facilitator and the focus group's reaction to the two styles of contemporary Child Care Licensing regulations are found in Appendix IV of this book. (Note: At the time of this study, sections 745.8601 and 745.8403 were current and written in the Plain English style. Sections 725.2038 and 725.2001 are in the traditional legalese style and were recently repealed.)

    A.

        RULE §725.2038. Notification of Non-compliance. The facility is entitled to written notification of any non-compliance with the conditions of probation or evaluation, including non-compliance with standards and/or the law.

        Source: Texas Administrative Code: Title 40 Social Services and Assistance, Part 2. West Group, 2001.

    B.

        RULE §745.8601 What happens if I am deficient in a minimum standard, rule, law, specific term of my permit, or condition of evaluation, probation, or suspension?

We may make recommendations and/or impose remedial actions for any deficiency.

Source: Office of the Texas Secretary of State. Texas Administrative. Title 40 Social Services and Assistance, Part 19, Chapter 745, Subchapter K, Division 1. Section. 745.8601. (2005a).

C.

RULE §745.8403 What is the purpose of an inspection?
The purpose of an inspection is to:

(1) Verify compliance with licensing statutes, rules, and minimum standards;
(2) Assess the risk to children in facilities;
(3) Evaluate whether the operation is subject to regulation;
(4) Assist the provider in identifying problems contributing to violations of licensing statutes, rules, and minimum standards;
(5) Offer technical assistance; and
(6) Gather information as part of an investigation.

Source: Office of the Texas Secretary of State. Title 40 Social Services and Assistance, Part 19, Chapter 745, Subchapter L, Division 1. Section. 745.8403. (2005b)

D.

RULE §725.2001. Inspection Visits. Unregulated and regulated facility/ registered/ or listed home staff must admit licensing staff and not delay or obstruct licensing staff from making inspections during hours of operation.

(1) Although the licensee/registrant/listee of a regulated facility may choose to limit children to certain areas of the structure, the licensee/ registrant/listee must allow the licensing representative to inspect any area of the facility/registered or listed family home that affects or could affect the health, safety, or well-being of the children in care. When inspection is refused, obstructed, or delayed by facility/registered or listed family home staff to the extent that licensing staff cannot carry out their responsibility, the facility/registered or listed family home shall be advised that these actions are in violation of the Human Resources Code, §42.044(a), and that the license/certificate/registration/listing may be revoked and/or legal action requested if resistance continues.

(2) More than one inspection visit may be necessary to complete an investigation or make a determination of compliance with licensing rules and standards.

Source: Texas Administrative Code: Title 40 Social Services and Assistance, Part 2. West Group, 2001.

THE FOCUS GROUP IN CONTEXT

In *On the Sublime,* Longinus wrote, "The term image in its most general acceptation includes every thought, howsoever presented, which issues speech. But the term is now generally confined to those cases when he who is speaking, by reason of the rapt and excited state of his feelings, imagines himself to see what he is talking about and produces a similar illusion in his hearers" (1952, p. 103). In the focus groups, the participants who read the regulatory text imagined government personnel as "stuffed shirts" with cattle prods, saw drop-down menus that led to nowhere, and visualized images of Communist Russia. Did these images lead focus group members to believe the worst of government inspectors and writers? Was it because of these images that emerged from the text that the focus group members assumed that the regulations are "overapplied" to African Americans? In this section, I will try to contextualize what the focus group members saw when they read the Plain English and legalese versions of the Child Care Licensing regulations. In the text, the focus group members saw (1) "wordiness" or unnecessary detail, (2) ambiguity, (3) abstract language, (4) discriminatory language, (5) participation in rule writing, (6) clarity, (7) punitive language, (8) comprehensiveness, (9) flexibility, (10) uncooperative language, and (11) cooperative language. These are the issues that the focus group members stressed when discussing the pros and cons of the two major styles of regulatory writing.

Stella Ting-Toomey suggests that in some cultures, wordiness in written contracts evokes distrust (1999, p. 223). In A Plain English Handbook: How to Create Clear SEC Documents, by the Office of Investor Education and Assistance, one means listed for making government discourse more concise is to delete "unnecessary details" (Securities and Exchange Commission, p. 17). When I asked the focus group members which regulations were easiest to read, they engaged in the following conversation:

> Subject A: "Rule B is easier to understand because it was expressed in everyday language as if the person was speaking with us."
>
> Subject F: "Rule A was because it is the opposite [of what of Subject A stated] because it does not speak directly to you but it is in a standard format that is easier to understand."
>
> Subject D: "Rule B because it is straightforward and says what would happen if it were to take place."
>
> Subject B: "Rule A because I had to drop out some words that I thought were unnecessary to understand B."
>
> Subject C: "Rule B because it is in laymans terms and plain language because you wouldn't have to guess about what a word means."

One focus group participant suggested that he needed to "drop out" some words to understand the question portion of the question-and-answer portion of Rule B, Section 745.8601, a Plain English regulation. Another preferred the legalese style used in Rule A, Section 725.2028 because this participant was familiar with the legalese style. Other participants said they preferred the Plain English regulation because it was "expressed in everyday language" or "layman's terms." Regarding Rule D, Section 725.2001, written in the legalese style, one participant stated, "Every one of those words in D with a slash has a drop down screen that seems like they link to some other catch. Rules are linked and you have to have a battery of, not one, lawyers to defend yourself and even they have problems. Attorneys still have problems; what chance do black people have to overcome legalese?" The hypertext analogy is powerful in that the participant proposes that the rule as written on the page does not stand alone, but it is connected to several other rules or "catches" that the audience cannot find. This analogy describes an endless number of hyperlinks leading to different Web pages, none of which contain the needed information. Another concern was the use of slashes in words like "unregulated and regulated facility/registered or listed home." The focus group members were confused by regulations without definitions. The group paid especially close attention to section 725.2001 and its reference to "unregulated and regulated facility/registered or listed home," which led to a long discussion about what these terms meant and why they were included.

> Subject B: "Words like "unregulated/regulated" allows for ambiguity and that in itself tends to leave open some kind of action. It tends to lean toward the agency. All of the slashes seem to make it seem like there is no end to it. As a layperson, I think it is poorly written. An attorney might say that it is a great rule."
>
> Subject C: "Unregulated" lets me know that if my business is unregulated that I shouldn't be in business. How can you function as an unregulated facility?"
>
> Subject B: "Define 'obstruct.' Anything that looks as if they don't want to define what is it makes it unclear."
>
> Subject F: "Words are definable; it just depends on who defines it. This leaves the door wide open for interpretation."
>
> Subject C: "The whole regulation D is written to oppose you. Why would an unregulated facility be mentioned?"
>
> Subject D: "I operate both an unregulated and a regulated facility and you're better off to operate a regulated facility and let them in. In an . . . facility you don't have to apply for a license, but someone in the community

may report you thinking you're supposed to be regulated and they come out to inspect . . . to make sure that you're out of compliance even though you're not supposed to be regulated. They look at the number of . . . I'm licensed for in the regulated facility. So my licensed facility hinges on my unregulated facility. Are there regulations for regulated and unregulated?"

Subject C: "They have a way to get you no matter what—even if you don't let them in because you're unregulated. Wow!" [The group laughs.]

Subject B: "In daycare centers, it's my understanding that once you're licensed, you're unregistered or listed. There are still regulations for all types of daycare facilities."

Most of the group thought the Plain English Rule C, Section 725.8403 was easier to understand than the legalese Rule D, Section 725.2001, because the Plain English version did not discuss an unregulated facility. There was still confusion about what an "unregulated facility" is and why it is mentioned if unregulated facilities are exempt from regulation. To remedy this type of confusion, the authors of *A Plain English Handbook: How to Create Clear SEC Documents* recommend that writers provide their audience with some background information before presenting new information and suggest the use of a question-and-answer format to make abstract terms concrete (Securities and Exchange Commission, 1998, pp. 23, 29). While focus group participants were concerned with ambiguous terms in both styles of regulation, they praised the Plain English regulations "as if the person was speaking with us" and as having a helpful tone.

Subject C: "All of the language in the first regulation [Section 745.8403] seems helpful. It's my business and you laid it out for me so that I can keep my business in compliance."

Subject B: "The first regulation lists everything that needs to be listed— "assist," "compliance," "offer assistance," "information.""

Subject A: "The second regulation [Section 725.2001] tells you what they are going to do with you and for you; it introduces their job title to you."

Subject F: "The first one is clear. C [Section 745.8403] covers everything that D [Section 725.2001] is saying and C seems helpful in nature."

Subject B: "The first one [Section 745.8403] sounds like I'm going to do this for you. Two [Section 725.2001] sounds like I'm going to do it *to* you as many times as possible."

Subject B: "Rule D leaves a lot of room for personalities to show their heads. "And/or" and "resistance" sound as if it is your mother pointing her finger at you. Resistance is futile, and I'm coming at you. The first line, they refer to "refusal" before anyone even said they would refuse it." [The group laughs.]

In their explanation of how trust and equal treatment are intertwined, Aberbach and Walker (1970) quote from George Sabine's "The Two Democratic Traditions," (p. 1199). The authors argue "The existence of distrustful citizens who are convinced that the government serves the interest of a few rather than the interests of all is a barrier to the realization of the democratic ideal." The statements recorded by focus group members certainly support Sabine's argument. The African American business owners reached a quick consensus when asked if government regulations were applied differently to African American business owners. When I asked the focus group, "Do you believe that the way regulations are written may contribute to this trust or are there other factors," three subjects engaged in the following conversation, which suggests that these business owners view rules that allow "wiggle room" as rules that evoke distrust in African American business owners because these are the rules that allow discrimination in their application.

> Subject B: "Not that African Americans don't understand the rules. We have to look at the history and how they've been changed and modified. Since slavery ended, we've learned how to play the rules, and they overlook the rules, don't play by them, or change them. They will boldface ignore what the rule says."
>
> Subject D: "I try to look at it as being applied as equally across the board knowing that's not true. We were able to get enough facility owners to get the State to get a standard where all of the inspectors are trained to look at the same things when they came out, and we were effective in getting that done. They would come in my place and look at certain things and go somewhere else look at other things. Now they use a checklist. The enforcement of rule is misapplied."
>
> Subject F: "It is the way the rule is written that gives them the leeway to misapply the regulation."
>
> Subject B: "Then we have to go back and show how it was misapplied. We're fighting the same battle we've been fighting for a hundred years, and most of the time it's overapplied on us."

Hagner and Pierce argued that the Civil Rights movement had caused blacks to form a strong group political identity that was not inherent in other ethnic or racial groups (Howell & Fagan, 1988, p. 346) At one point in the focus group meeting, when I asked if everyone agreed with a prior statement and one focus group member replied, "We're all black aren't we?" he made an argument that many would view as indicative of a monolithic or essentialized view of African Americans and African American perceptions. Although African Americans have never been a monolithic group who shared the same ideals and values, as was so eloquently expressed in Dubois' *The Souls of Black Folks,* contemporary

African Americans' shared history, knowledge of past discriminatory laws and practices, and group political identity help shape their perceptions. In "Race, Representation, and Trust: Changes in Attitudes After the Election of a Black Mayor," the authors used quantitative research methods to compare political trust levels in African American and white Americans in 1970 and 1976 and found that trust levels were linked to African American's perception of black participation in policy development (Abney & Hutcheson, 1981, p. 93). The focus group members' belief in the importance of African American participation in regulation development as a means of evoking trust is clear in the following exchange:

> Subject F: "I didn't know that they did that kind of research. Both, the way regulations are written does contribute to this fact. Are African Americans involved in writing regulations in the first place? Does anyone know of a black regulation writer?"
>
> [No one responded.]

Trudy Glover argues, "When we trust others, we expect them to act in ways that are helpful, or at least not harmful to us. We have a sense that they are persons of integrity, persons capable of reliable action, persons well motivated, with proper concern and respect for others" (1992, p. 17). The subjects pointed out that in one legalese regulation, the writer began with a punitive tone, which sounded as if the government accused the business owner before providing any context for the fines or punishment. Many of the focus group members believe that regulatory agents have a personal interest in finding noncompliances or rule violations when inspecting or evaluating their businesses. One subject stated,

> Government regulators or enforcers are motivated by how many fines they can place on you. They are bonused by how many fines they can place on you. I can imagine that daycare facilities and home health care facilities are bonused on how many they can get. The people who write these rules are trying to help the enforcers get these bonuses.

Although there is no evidence to support this claim, the suggestion that regulation-enforcement staff have a vested interest in citing the regulated entities for noncompliances with State regulations demonstrates an obvious lack of trust in enforcement practices and the *ethos* of government agencies.

The focus group members were particularly bothered by the language in the Child Care Licensing's repealed Section 725.2001, which begins with "Inspection Visits" (Texas Administrative Code, 2001). "Unregulated and regulated facility/registered/ or listed home staff must admit licensing staff and not delay or obstruct licensing staff from making inspections during hours of operation." The focus group proposed that beginning a regulation with words suggesting what a regulated entity might do wrong assumes the worst of the business owner. The business owners preferred the language used in Plain English Rule C, Section 745.8403, which begins by situating the audience with a question and reads, "What is the purpose of an inspection? The purpose of an inspection is to:" (Office of Texas Secretary of State, 2005b). The focus group preferred Plain English Rule C, Section 745.8403 because it outlined the requirements without beginning the regulation with images of negative actions on their part and punitive actions by the government.

Still, one participant preferred the legalese styled Rule D, Section 725.2001 because it identified the actor; Subject A stated, "The second regulation tells you what they are going to do with you and for you; it introduces their job title to you." In Chapter II of this book, I argue that although it is important to assess the *ethos* of the author, it is just as important to evaluate the enforcement and authoritative figures invoked in the actual text of the regulations to ascertain what Texas freed blacks must have thought, not of those writing the regulations, but those images or characters invoked in the regulations. Subject A wanted to know the person evaluating her business and their title. This same subject stated that the legalese version "tells you what they are going to do with you and for you." Another subject argued that the Plain English Rule C, Section 745.8403 covered the same issues addressed in the legalese Rule D, Section 725.2001, but in a "clear" and "helpful nature."

On the other hand, uncooperative language would likely be received as examples of "harmful" actions that regulated entities or persons could face (Glover, 1992, p. 17). The focus group members argued that the legalese regulation seemed to be "written to oppose you" or was uncooperative. One participant stated that while the Plain English Rule C, Section 745.8403, "sounds like I'm going to do this for you," the legalese version suggested that "I'm going to do it *to* you as many times as possible." It was obvious that the focus group members viewed the legalese version as harmful and, according to Glover, more likely to evoke distrust. Glover simply suggests that we trust people who want to help or cooperate with us (p. 17). Overall, the focus group members' responses recommend the tone of the Plain English regulations, especially the use of first-person and the question-and-answer format. The participants viewed these regulations not only as legal requirements but also as technical assistance or help, which Glover believes evokes trust in audiences (p. 17). One participant confirmed that the Plain English version evoked trust and stated, "It makes me more trustful," while another stated, "The tone in B [Plain English Section 745.8601] opens up with a question that makes you feel better about the rule and even acknowledge that you may be deficient and that they are willing to work with you."

These focus group members' comments suggested that they do understand the rule writer's need for flexibility in style and language. The focus group members' assessment is consistent with my argument in Chapter I of this book, when I reviewed the classical rhetoricians' ideas about style and regulatory discourse; their arguments about the appropriate rhetorical strategies were very much dependent on the rhetorical situation, as is most persuasive discourse. With any real attention to contexts, there is an implied recognition of the need for flexibility or stylistic choice. The focus group members' acceptance of the need for some flexibility in style is also in line with one policy writer, who stated, "They can't have it both ways, clarity and objectivity." With each regulation, the policy writer certainly needs flexibility to make stylistic trade-offs, depending on their various goals and audiences.

In the next and final chapter, I make recommendations for the use of a plain style of regulatory writing, which considers the needs of the user as well as the audience, whether this audience is invoked or addressed. I make recommendations for stylistic and linguistic choices that promote trust in historically marginalized groups, with the hope that these efforts will evoke trust in this and a broader, less skeptical audience. Finally, I synthesize the results of all of the case studies in this book into an invention heuristic for regulatory writing that addresses distrustful audiences.

CHAPTER VI

An Invention Heuristic for Regulatory Writing

In December 1999, while I was working as the Rules Coordinator for the Child Care Licensing Rule Review, the Division Administrator asked me to give a speech during an annual training meeting for our field staff, who were gathering from around the state. My task was to explain the definition of rules and the new law that required the agency to review rules. In the speech, as a joke, I mentioned that those of us in the rulemaking office would appreciate it if the field staff would forgo their rights to make public comments. The joke was well received by this audience because field staff rarely made public comments anyway. In reality, this audience was made up of administrators and inspectors from around the state who were privy to the internal drafts of proposed regulations because each Child Care Licensing Office, whether located in Houston, Dallas, Lubbock, San Antonio, or Austin, had regional administrators who had face-to-face access to Child Care Licensing policy writers at least once a month. The field staff, my audience, made comments weekly to their administrators, who in turn made comments directly to the writers. For the most part, their voices were heard and often impacted rulemaking, and even initiated it.

A few months later, I was asked to give a similar speech to the Child Care Licensing Advisory Board, which was made up of a group of childcare providers and childcare advocates. In this meeting, in lieu of the joke that I mentioned above, I stressed the importance of their feedback and input in the Division's rule review process. I also welcomed public comments and informed them that their comments would be published in the *Texas Register* for all to see. My reason for choosing not to joke about the advisory board and other business owners' right to participation in rule development should be obvious; in our country, "the public" has often had to fight for fair representation and the acknowledgement of their voices in the promulgation of laws and even regulations. Thus, even a joke about refusing them access to this vital process, which affects their children and businesses, could likely evoke distrust. As in any rhetorical situation, where persuasion is the aim, I considered my audience, their possible responses, and the *ethos* of my agency and myself.

I am certain that many readers of this study might ask themselves, "where do we draw the line?" when considering people's emotional responses and our own *ethos*. And my response is the same as when I am asked this question by my undergraduate students who argue that Mike Markel's calls for clear safety instructions in his textbook, "Technical Communication" is "dumbing down" our society (Markel, 2004, p. 523). One student stated that if a reader can't understand safety manual instructions and engages in dangerous and unsafe behavior because the reader can't understand complex words, it's simply a case of "survival of the smartest." The student, a science major, was making a rational argument based on his preference for efficiency over equality (I mention this ongoing argument about equality versus efficiency in my discussion of Okun's 1975 work in Chapter II of this book). In an attempt to appeal to this student's preference for efficiency, where the writer does not take the time to consider an uneducated audience, I asked the student about the purpose of the instruction manual. Why does the company produce a safety manual? I asked the student about the writer's desired ends. The student agreed that the writer's goal was to make sure that the reader was not harmed physically, so it would be reckless for the writer to continue to use terms that someone who isn't "smart" would not understand. As technical communicators, when dealing with issues—beyond clarity, brevity, and sincerity—we can use the line of reasoning of my undergraduate and argue that it would be reckless for us to fail to consider historical texts and contexts that impact our audience when writing for audiences who still remember these texts and contexts. It would be irresponsible for us to disregard knowledge bases that can help us to persuade an audience, even if we don't see the validity of their complaints. The contextual inquiry and focus group portions of this study reveal that the African American audience is still skeptical of government regulations, and policy writers are aware of minority distrust. Both groups believe that the Plain English style can help to increase trust in government regulations.

IMPLICATIONS OF CONTEXTUAL INQUIRY AND FOCUS GROUP STUDIES

In the United States, a society where people of all ethnicities and races own businesses and all are required to comply with regulations, regulatory writers must acknowledge that there is a need for the employment of rhetorical strategies; there is a need for persuasion. If Plain English regulations evoke trust in African American audiences that have been historically disenfranchised, this trust may be a step toward intercultural negotiation, which might transform into participation in rulemaking and increased compliance. With this said, I will now move into a discussion that explains what cultural factors are considered in regulatory writing (see Table 6.1).What style of regulatory writing meets the demands of the government agency as well as a distrustful African American audience?

Table 6.1 unveils those cultural factors that regulatory writers considered in drafting Child Care Licensing regulations. Although the writers' initial responses suggested that they were not very concerned about the ethnicity of their audience, Table 6.1 suggests that writers at Child Care Licensing considered more cultural variables than those black business owners at the focus group meeting anticipated. In the historical case study of the Texas Black Codes, the freedmen represented the audience who could not read or protect their own rights. In contemporary regulations, the literacy of business owners who do not speak or read English as their first language, and the children and elderly who cannot read but are protected by regulations, should be considered in regulation invention. One writer mentioned the fact that she wrote criminal background-check regulations, which disproportionately affected minorities, and another mentioned the fact that some Latinos who own registered family homes cannot read English. Another writer mentioned that she considered the voices of children as her

Table 6.1. Cultural Factors Considered in Regulatory Writing

Cultural factors	Did the CCL policy writers consider these cultural factors when writing regulations?	Style suggested by participants
Ethnic minorities	Yes	Plain English
Gender	No	Not addressed
Age—children and elderly who protect their rights	Yes	Not addressed
Geographic areas with increasing numbers of business owners who don't speak or read English	Yes	Plain English
Disabled (can't speak for themselves)	Yes	Plain English
Business owners with less than a GED or High School Diploma	Yes	Plain English
Literacy—Audiences who can't read the regulations	Yes	Not addressed

invoked audience, and the other writer suggested that education was an important cultural factor. All of the writers suggested that Plain English was the most appropriate style of writing to address the needs of their audience. Although the policy writers acknowledged that most Texas childcare providers are white women within a specific age group, the writers did not mention any cultural consideration that should be made for this particular audience.

In addition to providing answers to my research questions, the contextual inquiry study revealed responses to important questions that new employees need to know when first hired as regulatory writers and agreed that there is no official training for policy writers. So, in my discussion with this particular group of policy writers about cultural factors and regulatory writing style, they thought it just as important to discuss the following issues with new policy writers.

WHAT INFORMATION DO NEW POLICY WRITERS NEED TO KNOW?

- What are rules?
- How do agencies make rules?
- What are important rule writing tasks?
- What happens to agency knowledge when rule writers or decision makers leave?
- How do agencies make new rules consistent with laws and rules that are enforced by other agencies?
- How do agencies decrease duplication in rules?
- Who is the author of the rule?
- Which style of rule writing is effective?
- How do rule writers conduct research?
- How do rule writers use research to support policy changes?
- What are some innovations in rulemaking?

To help government agencies educate their staff, graduate programs in Technical Communication, Composition and Rhetoric, and Public Administration should consider developing regulatory or governmental writing courses. A rigorous approach to regulatory writing at the graduate level would prepare future policy writers for this very complex and important work.

In addition to addressing "What do New Policy Writers Need to Know?" students who enroll in a regulatory writing course should understand the place of public discourse in history and how historical events helped shape our current styles of writing. Many of the documents explored in a regulatory writing course will be unfamiliar to students who expect to work in government agencies, but an understanding of the theories that lead to effective technical communication on Web sites, reports, proposals, policy and procedures manuals, and document design would be useful as students begin to examine regulation preambles, legislative impact statements, public comments to proposed regulations, advocacy group Web sites, federal and state laws that prescribe regulations, and new e-rulemaking Web sites that allow citizen interaction with regulatory writers.

Since few technical documents address an audience as diverse as the public policy audience, it would not be difficult to ensure that students, in addition to exploring various types of discourse surrounding and including regulatory writing, also pay close attention to the multicultural audiences that contribute to the invention of regulatory discourse. Incorporating an examination of multicultural audiences is, again, an attempt to address the need that scholars in technical communication have identified. Over 10 years ago, Susan Mallon Ross reported, "a random survey of members of the Society of Technical Communication [$N = 63$], on average, rated study of intercultural communication by technical communication students as 'nice, but not necessary' (1994, p. 473)." The recent increase in the number of intercultural technical communication scholarly articles and courses proves that this perception is changing. Still, I would argue that many graduate-level courses in technical communication address genres of technical communication (proposals, reports, manuals, online publications) that are far less appropriate for thorough examinations of variations in the responses of multicultural audiences within the United States than regulatory writing. My argument is based on the fact that regulations address broad audiences that include ethnic minorities and have a history of evoking emotions that make these artifacts more susceptible to divergent responses. So, as graduate students explore regulations and the audiences that affect the invention of regulations, some discussion of the contexts in which these texts are produced and the cultures of these audiences must be explored.

Classroom discussions of assigned readings and activities should do more than discuss style and document design of rules and their accompanying documents (memos, derivation tables, fiscal impact statements, etc.), but discuss "whose interests are protected and reproduced through community norms"(Thralls & Blyler, 1993, p. 254). Charlotte Thralls and Nancy Roundy Blyler position these types of classroom activities and assignments under a liberatory pedagogy embraced by James Berlin, Patricia Bizzell, and Carolyn Miller, whose insights have been influenced by Jurgen Habermas, Michel Foucault, and Paulo Freire (Thralls & Blyler, 1993, p. 253).

WHAT STYLE MEETS THE NEEDS OF THE GOVERNMENT AGENCY AND THE PUBLIC?

The analysis of the data collected from the policy writers and business owners reveals that all participants, writers and audiences, prefer the Plain English style of writing. Both groups believe that Plain English regulations evoke trust and are clear and also believe that legalese is difficult to understand and more likely to evoke distrust. Still, proponents of the Plain English movement must realize that the use of the Plain English style alone does not respond to my question regarding historically marginalized groups. My discourse analysis of Texas Black Codes in Appendices I and II makes it obvious that translations from legalese to Plain English without consideration of trust-related issues and the past relationship between some historically marginalized business owners and the government does nothing to evoke trust. As you will see in these Appendices, Plain English versions of the Texas Black Codes were just as sinister as the legalese versions. When dealing with historically marginalized groups, the Plain English version of regulations must tell the whole story; it must be comprehensive, because this group is most distrustful of regulations that are not comprehensive. The contemporary African American business owners who participated in my study want to know who is being addressed, who isn't being addressed, who is enforcing the regulation, who isn't enforcing the regulation, the definitions of words, and the exclusion of words that have no direct affect on the regulation. This distrustful audience wants nondiscriminatory regulations, comprehensiveness, brevity, clarity, concrete terms, cooperative tone, and evidence of participation in rule-making; they even acknowledged the need for rule writers to have some flexibility. They believe that if they know what they are expected to do, there is a decreased chance that they will be treated differently or unfairly.

In 1866, regulatory writing by members of the 11th Texas Legislature was carried out by state legislators who wrote laws regulating black labor without interference from any state or local government and with blatant disregard for the input from the federal agency charged with oversight of black labor. In my examination of the invention and enforcement of the 11th Texas Legislature's Black Codes, I found no evidence of an open regulation development process where the regulated entities were allowed to express their opinions of the regulations or even read them. There is no evidence of participation in regulatory development. So, if interested parties had no opportunity to comment on or even read the regulations prior to codification, it is not surprising that writers of Texas Black Codes, who were accustomed to using the legalese style, did not use a plain style to appeal to their audience, especially since the intent of the Texas Black Codes conflicted with federal law and ethical behavior. The 11th Texas Legislative Session's closed regulatory writing process was quite different than our current regulatory writing processes where *writers,* not elected legislators, are asked to follow the processes similar to what Child Care Licensing policy writers call a "rule development process." In technical communication, we would very likely refer to any process consisting of these important elements—write, feedback, edit, approve, and implement—as a collaborative writing process. Any process, so filled with revision, research, internal and external notification, collaboration, and approval is open, and this openness demands a more credible style of writing. With this new and open system, African American business owners as well as other historically marginalized groups can impact the intent and language of regulations.

Now, so many years after Texas' Black Codes, we have African American business owners interested in whether or not a small state childcare licensing agency has any African American rule writers and who admit that the Plain English style (because of its clarity, concrete terms, and brevity) makes them more trustful, but who are still cognizant and wary of the potential for discrimination in the application of any style of regulatory discourse. Regardless of the style, these African American business owners are sensitive to excessively punitive language, want comprehensive regulations, desire a cooperative tone, and yet, can still acknowledge the rule writer's need for flexible rules that account for contingencies and organizational norms.

Now, so many decades since legislators wrote labor regulations without the help of agencies, we have policy writers who claim that they consider the voices of historically marginalized groups when writing regulations. In some cases, the policy writers themselves are minorities and women who might be sensitive to and cognizant of language or a style that evokes distrust. We have policy writers who will admit a preference for writing in the legalese style because Plain English requires more thought, more skill, and more contexts, but still advocate the plain style because it is what the audience needs. And, in my discussions with policy writers, we find that they too have needs, from both industry and academia, to write effective regulations. Policy writers, who are seldom students of technical communication or composition and rhetoric, need to understand the various writing processes involved in their work as well as the very nature of their work. The writers suggest that new policy writers need to know what rules are, circumstances under which rules are written, how to be consistent in rules and laws, how to maintain institutional knowledge when personnel change and tacit and historical knowledge are lost, what innovations are being explored in rule writing, who the authors of rules are, how to conduct and defend research that supports rules, and common rule writing styles.

Toward this aim, I present a Rulemaking Heuristic, designed to evoke trust in a distrustful audience, that contains recommendations gathered from the historical and contemporary case studies as well as some of the policymaking and rhetorical theories presented in the literature review of this book. It is an attempt to synthesize what we know about rulemaking and how we can make it better, especially when translating regulations from the legalese style to the Plain English style. This heuristic can be used to facilitate policy writers interested in writing regulations that evoke trust not only in African American audiences but in our multiethnic and distrustful society. Based on the results of the historical discourse analysis of the Texas Black Codes, the contextual inquiry of State of Texas policy writers, and the focus group with African American business owners, regulation writers interested in evoking trust in distrustful audiences should consider the following before and during their writing process:

A RULEMAKING HEURISTIC TO EVOKE TRUST IN DISTRUSTFUL AUDIENCES

1. Acknowledge the writer's need to make a tradeoff between specific and broad terminology. Recognize the writer's role as advocate for the user as well as advocate for those whose interests are protected by the regulation. Thus, there are two sets of readers that the regulatory writer addresses, and while clarity protects those who need to comply with regulations, some level of vagueness in regulatory writing to account for contingencies might protect the interests of those protected by the regulation (see Figure 6.1).
2. Identify and document concerns of distrustful audiences (external stakeholders) that have a history of noncompliance or resistance to participation in regulation development.
3. Do not translate regulations from legalese to Plain English without reviewing the initial reason for adopting the regulation as well as the historical rationale for implementing it. In Appendices I and II, when important information was left out of the legalese version of the Texas Black Codes, the same information was left out of the Plain English translation. Without attention to the historical contexts in which regulations are written, regulatory writers will fail to include important information in Plain English regulations. To this end, writers must maintain and reference historical data.
    a. Create a digital record of internal and external documentation of discussions that affect these audiences. This record will help writers to make arguments for using specific language and tones when communicating with audiences. These audiences might be "addressed" (internal and external

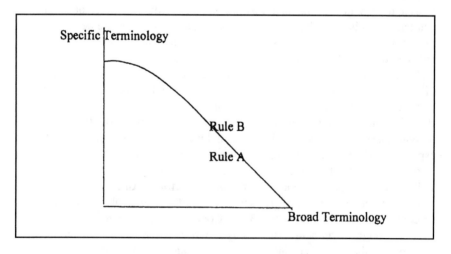

Figure 6.1. Negotiating rhetorical extremes.

stakeholders) or "invoked" (distrustful audiences, children, illiterates, stakeholders who cannot read, participants who do not participate but need the protection of regulations) (Ede & Lunsford, 1997, pp. 77–95).
   b. Consult historical data such as Council/Board memorandums, public comments, and disposition tables to better understand the historical contexts of similar regulations.
4. In addition to the Plain English rules or tips advocated by the Federal Government, regulation writers should consider the following criteria:
   a. In either the question or answer portion of the regulation, identify the intended audience. The Texas Black Codes were often written in passive voice and failed to identify the audience, making the regulation unclear and impersonal. In Appendices I and II, when these regulations are translated into Plain English, the audience is identified in the question portion of the regulation and addressed as "you" in the answer portion.
   b. Avoid the excessive use of slash marks. When reading the contemporary regulations, focus group members compared slash marks like "and/or" to drop-down menus on a computer interface that lead to never-ending requirements.
   c. Avoid repetitive prepositional phrases. In Chapter III, when comparing the *Texas Laws Made Plain* cotton baling regulations with those promulgated by the Texas Legislature in the early 1920s, it was obvious that redundant use of prepositional phrases is not necessary to communicate important information.
   d. Identify the job titles of the government staff responsible for inspecting or evaluating the regulated entity in the rule. Introduce the business owner to the inspector in the regulation; this is an effort at establishing a positive relationship. This proved effective in my Plain English translations of the Texas Black Codes in Appendices I and II. Also, a focus group member identified this strategy as trust-evoking in a contemporary legalese regulation written by the Child Care Licensing Staff (see Focus Group transcript in Appendix IV).
   e. Ambiguous and abstract terms in regulations can lead to inconsistency in the application of rules, which may be viewed by distrustful audiences as discriminatory. Thus, abstract terms and ambiguous regulations are not only confusing but potentially discriminatory if applied inconsistently. Follow the Child Care Licensing Division's rule of thumb of defining terms if the word has a different meaning in the dictionary.
   f. Do not hide the language that communicates important information in nonessential clauses. Do not subordinate the rights of some regulated entities. This strategy was often used in the Texas Black Codes and added to the deceptive nature of the codes.
   g. Use terms consistently throughout an entire rule section, chapter, and article. While the Texas Black Codes included language related to "costs"

88 / FROM BLACK CODES TO RECODIFICATION

and "fines" that were inconsistent with previous use, the Child Care Licensing policy writers stated that consistent language and content in their Plain English regulations was a goal.

h. Be especially cognizant of trust-related categories (see Table 2.1) when writing regulations that assign fines and punishment for noncompliance with regulations. Texas Black Codes that related to fines and punishments were blatantly discriminatory.

I. Do not reference other laws or statutes within regulations without identifying where these laws and regulations can be found. When Texas Black Codes referenced other laws without citing the law within the texts of the regulation, both the legalese and Plain English versions of the regulation were less clear.

j. Also, in documents that supplement regulations, like handbooks and manuals, it is important to reference the codified regulation so that audiences can be sure that the regulation still exists. In the *Texas Laws Made Plain* regulations, the apprenticeship codes did not reference any current law and included plain language versions of laws that had previously been repealed.

k. When clarity is the goal, avoid vague modifiers. Words like "moderate," "necessary," "proper," "suitable," "poor," and "competent" were used in Texas Black Codes to describe the degree of punishment that black minors could be subjected to and the removal of black minors from their households.

l. Consider the subject position that you assign your audience. The focus group members noted that the legalese regulations made them feel as if they were being chastised or dictated to. The Texas Black Codes include numerous examples of where the freed slaves were addressed without respect and as objects instead of contracting adults.

Figure 6.1 illustrates "the concept of scarcity and the consequent necessity to choose what to produce" (Knopf, 1991, pp. 244–245). The curve on the graph is a production-possibilities curve, which allows us to visualize our regulatory text and the dichotomous extremes we use to describe what we read. I believe that this illustration and its economic concept allows us to see the power the writer has (and should use) to move up and down that curve in an effort to balance their need or use of either clarity or vagueness, whichever is a priority in that particular situation. In the focus group meeting, one business owner stated, "Rule A is trying to be more inclusive of different things, and government regulations are usually more punitive because regulations are written to make a person do things. I can't see a government entity limiting itself the way B does." (See Figure 6.1 to demonstrate the focus group member's opinion about flexibility in rules versus clarity.) In this study, both regulatory writers and focus group members agreed that they need "flexibility" and that regulatory agencies could not "box themselves in." So, with each regulation, the writer is challenged with negotiating divergent aims—specific and broad terms, concrete and abstract terms, equality and efficiency, plain style and legalese style, reader goals and writer goals, negotiation and compliance—but with the acknowledgment of these areas where writers have flexibility to move along a production-possibilities curve, we must also acknowledge that there should be no compromises when dealing with trust in regulatory discourse, because even with the power the regulatory writers have and the limits in which they operate, they must be ever cognizant of the fact that regulatory writing can evoke trust.

While some focus group members understood the need for flexible regulations, they did not understand disrespectful tones or regulations with unnecessarily punitive tones. Even when there is a need to use abstract terms to give the agency flexibility to protect children or other invoked audiences who cannot ordinarily protect themselves, the writer can easily address the business owner in a cooperative and respectful tone. The writer must be certain that fines and punishments for noncompliance with regulations are determined and applied equally and consistently, and that the language used in regulations clearly represents what is possible in the real world. There should be an effort to be comprehensive and clear in explaining the context and scope of the regulation to the business owner so that even the business owner understands that the rule is broad in order to account for those unanticipated circumstances when they must be held accountable. In those circumstances where policy writers have no choice but to move closer to broadness/vagueness than specificity/clarity, they must make a special effort to be honest and use language and style that evokes trust.

CONSIDERATIONS FOR THE FUTURE OF REGULATORY WRITING

In a memorandum dated January 21, 2009, President Barack Obama wrote, "My Administration is committed to creating an unprecedented level of openness in Government. We will work together to ensure the public trust and establish a system of transparency, public participation, and collaboration (Obama, 2009, p. 4685). For the first time, calls for transparency in government are being heralded by an African American president, but residuals of distrust and lack of minority participation in regulation development persists. To combat government distrust and establish *ethos* across socioeconomic and ethnic lines, federal government agencies are designing technologies—electronic rulemaking—to overcome intercultural conflicts and provide new spaces for multiethnic democratic participation in regulation development on the Internet. While technological efforts to increase public participation in regulation development are indeed progressive, scholars in political science argue that the new method of participation will be hampered by the digital divide (Hague & Loader, 1999, p. 9).

Shulman, Scholosberg, Zavestoski, and Courard-Haruri (2003) define electronic rulemaking (e-rulemaking) as "a bridge from the first generation of Internet use—providing information to the public—to next generation: citizen to government commentary, and potentially citizen to citizen discourse, in the development of agency rules" (p. 1). While this reveals a divide between African Americans and rule writing processes, e-rulemaking has the potential to exacerbate this already tenuous relationship. While Shulman and colleagues explain that government agencies are prepared for public dissent against proposed rules and prepare rebuttals in the form of scientific evidence that minority audiences lack the social and economic capital to challenge, e-rulemaking does promise access to those citizens, including minorities, who may have greater access to rulemaking activities with e-rulemaking than without it (pp. 9–10). Adam Banks (2006) posits, "For material access to have any effect on people's lives or on their participation in the society, they must also have the knowledge and skills necessary to use those tools effectively" (p. 41). In e-rulemaking, the knowledge and skills required of citizens include the ability to comprehend the complex language of rules, keep abreast of evolving rule development processes, and navigate e-rulemaking Web sites. With e-rulemaking on the heels of the troublesome style of rules, scholars and practitioners in technical communication and rhetoric, public administration, political science, and human-computer interaction must identify and confront both the opportunity and challenge of this new technology. Opportunity lies in our willingness to consider the *ethos* of government agencies and make rhetorical choices to repair any harm that language contributes to distrust while we are still challenged to consider ways the e-rulemaking may help or hinder the access of minorities and the poor to rulemaking activities. Finally, Shulman and colleagues confess that "in an environment in which public trust of government officials and scientific experts at times appear to be broken down and where policy makers and agency personnel distrust citizen input, the public is unlikely to accept scientific justifications for a decision" (p. 10). With what we now know about African American distrust, its roots, and lingering fruit, we must be willing to confront the ways inaccessibility nurtures distrust in both language and technology. In contrast to classical rhetoric, which places the entire burden of proof on the rhetor through the establishment of their character, presentation of logical and trustworthy information, and appeals to the audience's emotions to move them in the "right" direction, scholars in African American rhetoric argue that at some point, the burden of proof shifts to the audience through "call and response, a reciprocal process" (Alkebulan, 2003, p. 37). Adisa A. Alkebulan argues that in the African oral rhetorical tradition "the absence of audience participation invalidates the event" (p. 37). Alkebulan's argument is consistent with experiences in the African American churches in the South, where a preacher might begin a sermon slowly and quietly with a presentation of the etymology of scripture and explanation of the historical and political contexts in which a selected scripture is written. But history has taught African Americans to be critical thinkers and to challenge ambiguity, so a pastor's use of classical Greek, a language foreign to most Americans, is only acknowledged with polite nods of the head and reluctant smiles. It is not until the pastor reaches a point of clarity and mentions information that the congregation knows to be true from their own study or experiences that someone will shout in encouragement and agreement, "Make it plain!" If regulatory agencies continue their attempts to "make it plain" in their use of language and technology, the African American audience will be encouraged to join in on regulatory discussions.

APPENDIX I

Texas Black Codes in Legalese and Plain English

THE RIGHTS OF "PERSONS OF COLOR"

CHAPTER CXXVIII.
An Act to define and declare the rights of persons lately known as Slaves, and Free Persons of Color.

Section 1. Be it enacted by the Legislature of the State of Texas, That all persons heretofore known as slaves, and free persons of color, shall have the right to make and enforce contracts, to sue and be sued, to inherit, purchase, lease, hold, sell, and convey real, personal and mixed estate; to make wills and testaments, and to have and enjoy the rights of personal security, liberty, and private property, and all remedies and proceedings for the protection and enforcement of the same; and there shall be no discrimination against such persons in the administration of the criminal laws of this State.

Sec. 2. That all laws and parts of laws relating to persons lately held as slaves, or free persons of color, contrary to, or in conflict with the provisions of this act, be and the same are hereby repealed; Provided, nevertheless, that nothing herein shall be so construed as to repeal any law prohibiting the intermarriage of the white and black races, nor to permit any other than white men to serve on juries, hold office, or vote at any election, State, county, or municipal; Provided further, that nothing herein contained shall be so construed as to allow them to testify, except in such cases and manner as is prescribed in the Constitution of the State.

Approved November 10, 1866.

Chapter CXXVIII
Source: University of North Texas Libraries: Gammel's Laws of Texas

CHAPTER CXXVIII.
Sec. 1. What are the rights of former slaves?
1. If you are a former slave, you have the right to enforce contracts, to sue and be sued, to inherit, purchase, lease, hold, sell, and transfer land, personal, and mixed property, to make wills and testaments, and have the right of personal security, liberty, private property, and all remedies and protections associated with these rights.
2. You will not be discriminated against in the enforcement of State of Texas criminal laws.

Sec. 2. What laws pertain to persons of color?
1. The Texas Legislature repeals all laws and parts of laws pertaining to freed slaves or freed persons of color that conflict with this chapter, except laws prohibiting the marriage of blacks and whites and laws prohibiting anyone other than white men to serve on juries, hold office, or vote in any state county or city election.
2. Recently freed slaves and free persons of color cannot testify in court except in cases mentioned in the Texas State Constitution.

Chapter CXXVIII in Plain English

DEFINING RACE AND RACE RELATIONS IN TEXAS

Article 34. All persons who have less than one-eighth African blood come within the meaning of the term "white persons," and all persons who have one-eighth, or a greater portion of African blood come within the meaning of the term "persons of color."

Article 408. If any person shall give, or barter, or cause to be sold, given or bartered, any ardent spirits, or any spirituous or intoxicating liquors, or fire arms, or ammunition to any Indian of the wild or unfriendly tribes, he shall be fined not less than ten nor more than one hundred dollars. Justices of the Peace and Mayors shall have jurisdiction under this article.

Articles 34 and 408
Source: University of North Texas Libraries: Gammel's Laws of Texas

CHAPTER LXXIII. Article 34. Who is considered a "person of color?"
Anyone with one-eighth or greater of African ancestry is a "person of color."
Anyone with less than one-eighth African ancestry is a "white person."

CHAPTER LXXIII. Article 408. May I conduct business with Indians?
If you give, trade, or sell any alcoholic beverages, or ammunition to any Indians

who are not allies of this state, you will be fined between ten and one-hundred dollars. Justices of the Peace and Mayors will enforce this article.

Article 34 and 408 in Plain English

VAGRANCY LAWS
CHAPTER CXL.

An Act to define the offence of Vagrancy, and to provide for the punishment of Vagrants:

Section 1. Be it enacted by the Legislature of the State of Texas, that a vagrant is hereby declared to be an idle person, living without any means of support, and making no exertions to obtain a livelihood, by any honest employment. All persons who stroll about to tell fortunes, or to exhibit tricks or cheats in public, not licensed by law, common prostitutes and professional gamblers, or persons who keep houses for prostitutes, or for gamblers; persons who go about to beg alms, (and who are not afflicted or disabled by a physical malady or misfortune); and habitual drunkards, who abandon, neglect or refuse to aid in the support of their families, and who may be complained of by their families; or persons who stroll idly about the streets of towns or cities, having no local habitation, and no honest business or employment, each and all of the above and aforesaid classes be, and they are hereby declared vagrants, coming with the meaning of this Act.

Sec. 2. The County Courts, Justices of the Peace, and Mayors or Recorders of incorporated towns and cities, shall have power to order the arrest of vagrants, and to try the offence provided for by this Act.

Sec. 3. A peace officer shall arrest a vagrant, and bring him or her before the Court or magistrate issuing the warrant, as herein provided for; and, if no peace officer can be conveniently procured, the warrant may be directed to any private person, who shall execute and return the warrant according to law.

Sec. 4. When a person arrested is brought before a court or magistrate, it shall be the duty of such court or magistrate to proceed to ascertain, by evidence, whether or not the accused is a vagrant within the meaning of this Act; and, if found guilty, he shall be fined in any sum not more than ten dollars.

Sec. 5. The accused shall, in every instance, if he demand it, be entitled to the right of trial by jury.

Sec. 6. In cases of conviction, the defendant shall not be released from custody until the fine and costs are paid; which, if not done within a reasonable time, to be judged of by the officer, the accused shall be put at such labor, and in such manner, as the Police Court of the county, or municipal authorities of towns and cities shall provide; and a vagrant who is so put to work, after conviction as aforesaid, shall not be released therefrom, until the fine and costs have been satisfied, at the rate of one dollar per day.

Sec. 8. A warrant may issue for the arrest of vagrants by the Judge of the County Court, or by a magistrate, and mayor or recorder, of their own motion, or on complaint, in writing, by some credible person, charging the offence.

Laws of the State of Texas.

Sec. 8. The Police Courts of the respective counties, and the municipal authorities of towns and cities, shall, at stated periods, make regulations prescribing the kind of work at which vagrants are to be employed. And should any vagrant refuse to work, after conviction and failure to pay fine and costs, he or she shall be lodged in jail, and placed in close confinement, on bread and water, until he or she may consent to work; and the period spent in jail shall not be computed in estimating the time for satisfying the fine and costs.

Sec. 9. Youthful and juvenile vagrants shall be sent before the Police Court, to be bound out, under the Act regulating Apprentices; Provided, that the fines and penalties prescribed in this Act shall conform to the provisions of the Criminal Code in relation to the same offences.

Sec. 10. All laws and parts of laws, in conflict with the provisions of this Act be, and the same are hereby repealed.

Approved November 8th, 1866.

Chapter CXI
Source: University of North Texas Libraries: Gammel's Laws of Texas

CHAPTER CXI.
Sec. 1. Who is considered a vagrant?
You are a vagrant if:
  a. You have no employment or means of financial support;
  b. You are an unlicensed fortune teller, trickster (con artist), cheat (swindler), prostitute, professional gambler, beggar (who is not ill or disabled), or drunkard (who is not providing financial support for your family);
  c. You are homeless and stroll the streets idly with no employment; or
  d. You provide shelter for prostitutes and professional gamblers.

Sec. 2. Who has the power to arrest and try a person for vagrancy?
The County Courts, Justices of the Peace, and Mayors or Recorders of incorporated towns and cities have the power to order the arrest of vagrants and try a person for vagrancy.

Sec. 3. Does a private citizen have the power to arrest a person suspected of vagrancy?
1. If you are a vagrant, a judge or magistrate may issue a warrant for your arrest.

2. A peace officer will arrest you and bring you before the court or magistrate who issued the warrant for your arrest.
3. If a peace officer is not available, a private citizen may arrest you and take you before the court or magistrate.

Sec. 4. What is the fine for vagrancy?
1. A judge or magistrate will evaluate evidence to determine if you are guilty of vagrancy.
2. If the judge or magistrate determines that you are guilty, you can be fined as much as $10.

Sec. 5. Do I have the right to request a trial by jury?
If you are accused of vagrancy, you have the right to request trial by jury.

Sec. 6. What happens if I am convicted of vagrancy?
1. If you are convicted of vagrancy, you will not be released from jail until you pay all costs and fines.
2. If you do not pay the costs and fines within a reasonable amount of time, the Police Court or municipal authorities in your jurisdiction will assign you to some labor.
3. The officer will decide how much time you have to pay the costs and fines before you are assigned to labor.
4. If you are convicted of vagrancy, you will not be released from labor until you pay all fines.
5. If you are convicted of vagrancy you will not be released from labor until you pay all fines, at the rate of one dollar per day.

Sec. 8 [Sec.7]. Who has the right to issue a warrant for a vagrant's arrest?
A County Judge, Magistrate, Mayor, Recorder, or credible citizen may issue a warrant to arrest a person for vagrancy.

Sec. 8. Who will decide what type of work vagrants perform?
1. The Police Courts and municipal authorities will make regulations that define the type of labor that convicted vagrants perform.
2. If you are a convicted vagrant and refuse to labor after failing to pay the costs and fines, you will be jailed in close confinement and fed bread and water until you agree to work.
3. The time that you spend in jail will not offset any fines or costs that you owe.

Sec. 9. What happens to juvenile vagrants?
1. If a juvenile is a vagrant, the juvenile will be apprenticed by the Police Court.
2. If the fines and penalties described in Chapter LXIII, An Act Establishing a General Apprentice Law and Defining the Obligations of Master and Mistress

and Apprentice are the same as those in the Criminal Code, the juvenile will be apprenticed under the apprenticeship guidelines in Chapter LXIII.

Chapter CXI in Plain English

CHAPTER LXIII.

An Act establishing a General Apprentice Law, and defining the obligations of Master and Mistress and Apprentice.

Section 1. Be it enacted by the Legislature of the State of Texas, That it shall be lawful for any minor to be bound as an apprentice, by his or her father, mother or guardian, with their consent, entered of record in the office of the Clerk of the county of which the minor is a resident, or without such consent, if the minor, being fourteen years of age, agree in open Court to be so apprenticed; Provided, There be no opposition thereto by the father or mother of said minor.

Sec. 2. It shall be the duty of all Sheriffs, Justices of the Peace, and other civil officers of the several counties of the State, to report to the Judge of the County Court of their respective counties, at any time, all indigent or vagrant minors, within their respective counties or precincts, and, also, all minors whose parent or parents have not the means, or who refuse to support said minors; and thereupon, it shall be the duty of the County Judge to apprentice said minor to some suitable and competent person, on such terms as the Court may direct, having particular care to the interest of said minor.

Sec. 3. All indentures of apprenticeship shall be approved by the County Judge, and entered of record in the office of the County Clerk of the county of which the minor apprenticed is a resident; and the County Judge shall have exclusive jurisdiction of all causes of action growing out of the relation of master or mistress and apprentice.

Sec 4. The term of apprenticeship of every minor, under this Act, shall be until the minor attains the age of twenty-one years, unless sooner married; Provided, that in all cases where the age of the minor cannot be ascertained by record, or other satisfactory testimony, the Judge of the County Court shall fix the same.

Sec. 5. It shall be the duty of the County Judge, upon making the order of apprenticeship, to require the master or mistress to give bond, in such sum as he may direct, with one or more good and sufficient sureties, payable to the County Judge and his successors in office, conditioned that he or she shall furnish said minor sufficient food and clothing—to treat said minor humanely—to teach or cause to be taught him or her some specified trade or occupation—to furnish medical attendance in case of sickness, and for the general and faithful compliance with the terms stipulated in the indentures as to education, &c.; and, in default of the master or mistress to comply with the stipulations of his or her bond, suit may be instituted by the father, mother or guardian of the minor, or by the County Judge, upon the same, for all damages sustained; and such damages, when recovered, shall be applied to the use and benefit of the apprentice, under such regulations as may be prescribed by the County Judge.

Sec. 6. That in the management and control of an apprentice, the master or mistress shall have power to inflict such moderate corporeal chastisement as may be necessary and proper.

Sec. 7. That if any apprentice shall run away from, or leave the employ of his master or mistress, without permission, said master or mistress may pursue and recapture said apprentice, and bring him before any Justice of the Peace of the county, whose duty it shall be to remand said apprentice to the service of his master or mistress; and, in the event of a refusal on the part of said apprentice to return, then the Justice shall commit said apprentice to the county jail, on failure to give bond for appearance, at the next term of the County Court; and it shall be the duty of the County Judge, at the next regular term thereafter, to investigate said cause, and, if the Court shall be of opinion that said apprentice left the employment of his master or mistress without good and sufficient cause, to order him to receive such punishment as may be provided by the vagrant laws then in force, until said apprentice agrees to return to his employment; Provided, That the Court may grant continuances, as in other cases; And further provided, That if the Court shall be of opinion that said apprentice has good cause to quit said employment, the Court shall discharge said apprentice from his indentures of apprenticeships.

Sec. 8. That in case any master or mistress of any apprentice may desire, he or she shall have the privilege to summon his or her apprentice to appear before the County Court of the county in which the parties may reside, and, on good and sufficient cause being shown to said Court, and on proof that said apprentice will not be injured thereby, shall be released from all liability, as master or mistress of such apprentice, and his bond canceled.

Sec. 9. It shall not be lawful for any apprentice, bound under the provisions of this Act, to reside out of the county, in the office of which, the terms of indenture are required to be recorded, without the written order of the County Judge, entered of record in the Clerk's office of the County Court of such county; when such leave is obtained, a certified copy of the order, authorizing the same, shall be filed for record in the office of the Clerk of the County Court of the county wherein the residence is to be; and the County Judge of that county shall have plenary power to hear and adjudicate all causes of action between the said master or mistress and apprentice, as fully as the County Judge of the County wherein the indentures of apprenticeship were originally recorded.

Sec. 10. Any apprentice who shall be removed out of the bounds of the county having original jurisdiction of the same, by his master or mistress, or with his knowledge or consent, without leave first obtained from the County Judge, and shall be retained thereout for a longer period than thirty days, shall not be held liable for a further compliance with his indentures, and can only be retained by the master or mistress at the pleasure of said apprentice.

Sec. 11. Any person who shall, knowingly and willfully, entice away an apprentice, or conceal or harbor a deserting apprentice, shall, upon conviction thereof, pay to the master or mistress, five dollars ($5.00) per day, for each day said apprentice is so absent, or concealed from his master or mistress, and shall likewise be held liable for all damages proved to have been sustained by the master or mistress, on account of such willful concealing, harboring, or enticing away, to be recovered by suit, before any Court having jurisdiction of the same.

Sec. 12. The County Judge shall have power to hear and determine and grant all orders and decrees, as herein provided, as well in vacation as in term time; Provided, That, in all applications for apprenticeship, ten days' public notice, as in case of guardianship, shall be given, and no minor shall be apprenticed except at a regular term of said Court.

Approved October 27, 1866.

Chapter LXIII
Source: University of North Texas Libraries: Gammel's Laws of Texas

CHAPTER LXIII.

Sec. 1. What consent is required to apprentice a minor?
1. A father, mother, or guardian must give consent to allow a minor to work as an apprentice.
2. A record of the father, mother, or guardian's consent must be filed with the county clerk in the county in which the minor lives.
3. If the minor is fourteen years old or older, the minor can agree in court to serve as an apprentice with the consent of a father, mother, or guardian.

Sec. 2. Who is responsible for identifying and reporting vagrants suitable for apprenticeship?
1. Sheriffs, Justices of the Peace, and other county civil officers must report indigent or vagrant minors and minors whose parents cannot support them to the County Judge.
2. The County Judge must apprentice minors who are indigent or vagrant to a suitable and competent citizen.
3. The court may set special restrictions for the terms for the apprenticeship to protect the minor.

Sec. 3. Who will approve and negotiate apprenticeships?
1. The County Judge will approve all apprenticeships.
2. The County Clerk will keep records of apprenticeships of minors in his or her county.
3. The County Judge will mediate all negotiations and conflicts between Masters, Mistresses and their apprentices.

Sec. 4. How long will a minor be apprenticed?
1. A minor will be apprenticed until the age of twenty-one or until married.
2. The County Judge will set the number of years of apprenticeship in cases when the minor's age is unknown or cannot be proven through records of court testimony.

Sec. 5. What are the responsibilities of the master and mistress?
1. If you are the Master or Mistress of an apprentice, you must follow your County Judge's orders regarding apprenticeship, including the payment of the bond.
2. The amount of the bond will be set by the judge.
3. As conditions of the bond, you must:
   a. Provide the apprenticed minor with sufficient food and clothing,
   b. Treat the apprenticed minor humanely,
   c. Teach the apprenticed minor a trade or make sure that another person teaches the minor a trade,
   d. Provide the minor with professional medical care when needed,
   e. Comply with all of the laws and requirements regarding educating indentures or, in this case apprentices.
4. If you default on any stipulations of your bond, the apprentice's father, mother, or guardian may sue you for damages. If damages are recovered, the damages will be used to benefit the apprentice as defined by the County Judge.

Sec. 6. Am I allowed to punish my apprentice?
If you are the master or mistress of an apprentice, you can inflict moderate corporeal punishment when necessary.

Sec. 7. What should I do if my apprentice runs away?
1. If you are the master or mistress of an apprentice, and the apprentice leaves your employment without permission, you may pursue or recapture the apprentice and bring the apprentice before any County Justice of the Peace.
2. The County Justice of the Peace will jail the apprentice until the next court date.
3. On the next court date, the County Judge will investigate the reason the apprentice left your employment.
4. If the County Judge determines that the apprentice left your employment without good cause, the apprentice will be punished under conditions written in the current vagrancy laws until the apprentice agrees to return to employment with their master or mistress.
5. If the County Judge determines that the apprentice had good cause for leaving your employment, the apprentice will be relieved of their obligations of apprenticeship.

Sec. 8. How do I release my apprentice from employment?
1. If you are a master or mistress of an apprentice, you may ask the County Judge to release your apprentice from employment.
2. You must provide proof that releasing the apprentice from employment will not cause the apprentice harm.

Sec. 9. Where can my apprentice reside?
1. If you are the master or mistress of an apprentice, your apprentice cannot reside out of the county in which the terms of apprenticeship were originally recorded without the County Judge's permission.
2. If you receive permission to reside with your apprentice outside of the county, you must notify the county clerk in your new county of residence.
3. The County Judge in your new county of residence will then be responsible for hearing and making decisions about any actions related to the apprenticeship.

Sec. 10. Can a Master or Mistress take an apprentice out of the county where the apprentice is employed?
If you are an apprentice and your Master or Mistress takes you out of the county where you were originally apprenticed without permission from the county judge for more than 30 days, then you are no longer required to fulfill the terms of your apprenticeship.

Sec. 11. What if I want to help an apprentice to leave their master or mistress?
1. If you encourage, hide, or harbor an apprentice who deserts their master or mistress, you must pay the master or mistress $5 for each day that the apprentice is absent or hidden from their master or mistress.
2. You are also liable for all damages suffered by the master or mistress during the apprentice's absence.
3. These damages must be recovered by lawsuit in a court that has jurisdiction over the apprenticeship.

Sec. 12. How do I apprentice a minor?
1. A minor cannot be apprenticed until a ten-day public notice is posted to obtain permission from guardians to approve apprenticeship before a County Judge.
2. A County Judge can approve apprenticeship applications, including the duration of the apprenticeship and vacation time.

Chapter LXIII in Plain English

CONTRACTS AND BLACK LABOR

CHAPTER LXXX.

An Act Regulating Contracts for Labor.

Section 1. Be it enacted by the Legislature of the State of Texas, That all persons desirous of engaging as laborers for a period of one year or less, may do so under the following regulations:

All contract for labor for a longer period than one month shall be made in writing, and in the presence of a Justice of the Peace, County Judge, County Clerk, Notary Public, or two disinterested witnesses, in whose presence the contract shall be read to the laborers, and, when assented to, shall be signed in triplicate by both parties, and shall then be considered binding, for the time therein prescribed.

Sec. 2. Every laborer shall have full and perfect liberty to choose his or her employer, but when once chosen, they shall not be allowed to leave their place of employment, under the fulfillment of their contract, unless by consent of their employer, or on account of harsh treatment or breach of contract on the part of the employer, and if they do so leave without cause or permission, they shall forfeit all wages earned to the time of abandonment.

Sec. 3. One copy of the contract, above provided for, shall be deposited with the Clerk of the County Court of the county in which the employer resides; and the Clerk shall endorse thereon, filed, giving the date, and signing his name officially; the contract then shall have the force and effect of an authentic act, and be conclusive evidence of the intent of the parties thereto; but all disputes arising between the parties shall be decided before a court of competent jurisdiction, and said court shall have power to enforce the same.

Sec. 4. The Clerk of the County Court shall enter, in a well bound book kept for that purpose, a regular and alphabetical index to the contracts filed, showing the name of the employer, and the employed, the date of filing, and the duration of the contract, which book, together with the contract filed, shall, at all times, be subject to the examination of every person interested, without fee. The Clerk shall be entitled to demand from the party filing such contract, a fee of twenty-five cents, which shall be full compensation of all services required under this Act.

Sec. 5. All labor contracts shall be made with the heads of families; they shall embrace the labor of all the members of the family named therein, able to work, and shall be binding on all minors of said families.

Sec. 6. Wages due, under labor contracts, shall be a lien upon one-half of the crops, second only to liens for rent, and not more than one-half of the crops shall be removed from the plantation, until such wages are fully paid.

Sec. 7. All employers, wilfully failing to comply with their contract, shall, upon conviction, be fined an amount double that due the laborer, recoverable before any court of competent jurisdiction, to be paid to the laborer; and any inhumanity, cruelty, or neglect of duty, on the part of the employer, shall be summarily punished by fines, within the discretion of the court, to be paid to the injured party; provided, that this shall not be so construed as a remission of any penalty, now inflicted by law, for like offences.

Sec. 8. In case of sickness of the laborer, wages for the time lost shall be deducted, and, when the sickness if feigned, for purposes of idleness, and also, on refusal to work according to contract, double the amount of wages shall be deducted for the time lost, and, also, when rations have been furnished, and should the refusal to work continue beyond three days, the offender shall be reported to a Justice of the Peace or Mayor of a town or city and shall be forced to labor on roads, streets and other public works, without pay, until the offender consents to return to his labor.

Sec. 9. The labor of the employee shall be governed by the terms stipulated in the contract; he shall obey all proper orders of his employer or his agent, take proper care of his work-mules, horses, oxen, stock of all character and kind; also, all agricultural implements; and employers shall have the right to make a reasonable deduction from the laborers' wages for injuries done to animals or agricultural implements committed to their care, or for bad or negligent work. Failing to obey reasonable orders, neglect of duty, leaving home without permission, impudence, swearing or indecent language to, or in the presence of the employer, his family or agent, or quarreling and fighting with one another, shall be deemed disobedience. For any disobedience, a fine of one dollar shall be imposed on, and paid by the offender. For all lost time from work hours, without permission from the employer or his agent, unless in case of sickness, the laborer shall be fined twenty-five cents per hour. For all absence from home without permission, the laborer shall be fined at the rate of two dollars per day; fines to be denounced at the time of the delinquency. Laborers will not be required to labor on the Sabbath, except to take necessary care of stock, and other property on the plantation, or to do necessary cooking or household duties, unless by special contract for work of necessity. For all thefts of the laborer from the employer, of agricultural products, hogs, sheep, poultry, or any other property of the employer, or wilful destruction of property, or injury, the laborer shall pay the employer double the amount of the value of the property stolen, destroyed or injured, one-half to be paid to the employer, and the other half to be placed in the general fund, provided for in this section. No live stock shall be allowed to laborers without the permission of the employer. Laborers shall not receive visitors during work hours. All difficulties arising between the employer and laborers, under this section, shall be settled, and all fines imposed by the former; if not satisfactory to the laborer, an appeal may be had to the nearest Justice of the Peace, and two freeholders, citizens, one of said citizens to be selected by the employer, and the other by the laborers; and all fines imposed, and collected under this section, shall be deducted from the wages due, and shall be placed in a common fund to be divided among the other laborers employed on the place at the time when their wages fall due, except as herein provided; and where there are no other laborers employed, the fines and penalties imposed shall be paid into the County Treasury, and constitute a fund for the relief of the indigent of the county.

Sec. 10. Laborers, in the various duties of the household, and in all the domestic duties of the family, shall, at all hours of the day or night, and on all days of the week, promptly answer all calls, and obey and execute all lawful orders and commands of the family in whose service they are employed, unless otherwise stipulated in the contract, and any failure or refusal by the laborer to obey, as herein provided, except in case of sickness, shall be deemed disobedience, within the meaning of this Act. And it is the duty of this class of laborers to be especially civil and polite to their employer, his family and guests, and they shall receive gentle and kind treatment. Employers, and their families, shall, after ten o'clock at night, and on Sundays, make no calls on their laborers, nor exact any service of them, which exigencies of the household or family do not make necessary or unavoidable.

Sec. 11. That for gross misconduct on the part of the laborer, such as disobedience, habitual laziness, frequent acts of violation of their contracts, or the laws of the State, they may be dismissed by their employer; nevertheless the laborer shall have the right to an appeal to a Justice of the Peace, and two freeholders, citizens of the county, one of the freeholders to be selected by him or herself, and the other by his or her employer, and their decision shall be final.

Sec. 12. That all laws and parts of laws contrary to or conflicting with the provisions of this Act be, and are hereby repealed, and that this Act take effect from and after its passage.

Approved November 1, 1866.

Chapter LXXX
Source: University of North Texas Libraries: Gammel's Laws of Texas

CHAPTER LXXX.

Sec. 1. How do a laborer and employee make a binding contract?
To make a labor contract binding, you must:
    a. Make the contract in writing,
    b. Make the contract in the presence of a Justice of the Peace, County Clerk, Notary Public, or two disinterested witnesses.
    c. Make certain that the contract is read to the laborer.
    d. Make sure that both the laborer and employee agree to the terms by signing the contract in triplicate.

Sec. 2. What are my rights as a laborer?
1. You have the right to choose an employer.
2. Once you have chosen an employer, you cannot leave their employment unless:
   a. You have fulfilled the terms of your contract, or
   b. Your employer does not follow the contract or treats your harshly.
3. If you leave without good cause or your employer's permission, you will forfeit all wages earned during your employment.

Sec. 3. Who keeps record of the contract and handles disputes after the contract is signed?
1. You must provide a copy of the contract to the County Clerk in the county where the employer resides.
2. The County Clerk must file, date, and sign their names to the contract to make the contract binding.
3. All disputes that arise between you and your employer or laborer will be decided in court in the county where the employer resides.

Sec. 4. How are labor contracts filed?
1. The County Clerk must maintain an alphabetical index of contracts in a well-bound book.
2. The index will include the name of the employer, the laborer, the date the contract is filed, and the duration of the contract.
3. The index and contract will be available for examination without charge by anyone interested.
4. The County Clerk can demand a fee of 25 cents from the person filing the contract.

Sec. 5. What members of a laborers' family are allowed to make contracts with employers?
1. You must make labor contracts with heads of families.
2. The contracts will apply to all members of the family who are able to work.
3. The contracts are binding on adult and minor family members.

Sec. 6. How will employers pay wages to laborers?
1. Laborers wages must include:
   a. Liens for rent and
   b. Liens for one-half of the crops.
2. Not more than one-half of the crops will be removed from the plantation until wages are paid.

Sec. 7. What happens if an employer violates the terms of a labor contract?
1. If you are an employer and convicted of willfully violating the terms of your contract, you will be fined double the wages you owe your laborer.
2. The Court in your jurisdiction will recover the wages for the laborer.
3. At the discretion of the court, you will be fined an amount, which will be paid to the laborer, for any inhumanity, cruelty, or neglect of duty.
4. Your payment of such fines will not count toward any other penalties you must pay for the same offenses.

Sec. 8. What happens when I am sick and unable to work for my employer?
1. If you are sick, your employer may deduct wages for the time you did not work.
2. If you are not sick but pretend to be sick to avoid work, your employer may deduct double the wages for time you did not work.
3. If you receive rations and continue to refuse work for more than three days:
   a. You will be reported to the Justice of the Peace or Mayor of your town or city.
   b. You will also be forced to labor on roads, streets, and other public works without pay until you agree to return to work for your employer.

Sec. 9. What must a laborer do to meet the requirements of a labor contract?
1. You must do the following:
   a. Obey all orders of your employer.
      I. You are disobedient if you fail to obey reasonable orders, neglect of duty, leave home without permission, lack caution, swear or use indecent language in the presence of the employer and his family or representatives, or quarrel and fight with one another.
      ii. You will be fined and must pay one dollar for any act of disobedience.
      iii. You will be fined twenty-five cents per hour for any work time lost as a result of you leaving home without permission.
      iv. You will be fined two-dollars per day for all absence from home without permission.
   b. Take proper care of your employer's work mules, horses, oxen, stock, and agricultural implements.
   c. Pay your employer double the amount for the value of property you steal or stock or agriculture you destroy or harm, one half of which will be paid to the employer and the other half to a general fund.
2. Employers have the right to:
   a. Deduct from your wages from injuries done to animals or agricultural implements in your care, bad or negligent work.
   b. Denounce fines at the time of delinquency.

c. Excuse laborers from work on Sundays except to:
      I. take care of stock and property on the plantation.
      ii. do necessary cooking or household duties, unless by special contract for work of necessity.
   d. Handle all difficulties arising between you and your employer.
      I. If you are not satisfied with your employer's decision or resolution, you can appeal to the nearest Justice of the Peace and two freeholders, citizens. One of the citizens must be selected by the employer and the other by you.
      ii. All fines imposed and collected during this section shall be deducted from wages due and placed in a general fund to be divided among the employer's other laborers when wages are due.
      iii. When there are no other laborers, fines will be paid to the County Treasury and set aside for indigents.
3. You cannot:
   a. Take live stock without your employer's permission.
   b. Receive visitors during work hours.

Sec. 10. What are the duties of laborers?
1. You must:
   a. Be available for various household duties at all times of the day and night and on all days of the week.
   b. Obey and execute all lawful orders and commands of the family in whose service they are employed, unless otherwise stipulated in the contract.
   c. Be especially civil and polite to your employer's family, guest, and treat them gently and kindly.
2. If you refuse to obey employer orders, except in the case of sickness, you shall be deemed disobedient within the meaning of this act.
3. Your employer and their family must not call you after ten o'clock at night or on Sundays, ask you for services, or visit your home, unless they need to.

Sec. 11. Can a laborer be dismissed by an employer?
1. Your employer can dismiss you from employment for gross misconduct including:
   a. disobedience,
   b. habitual laziness,
   c. frequent violations of your contract, and
   d. frequent violations of State of Texas laws.
2. You have the right to appeal the dismissal to the Justice of the Peace and two county citizens. You can select one of the citizens and the employer may select the other.
3. The Justice of the Peace and the two citizens will make the final decision about the dismissal.

Chapter LXXX in Plain English

EMPLOYING LABORERS OR APPRENTICES UNDER CONTRACT

CHAPTER LXXXII.

An Act to provide for the punishment of persons tampering with, persuading or enticing away, harboring, feeding or secreting laborers or apprentices, or for employing laborers or apprentices under contract of service to other persons.

Section 1. Be it enacted by the Legislature of the State of Texas, That any person who shall persuade, or entice away from the service of an employer, any person who is under a contract of labor to such employer, or any apprentice, who is bound as such, from the service of his master, or who shall feed, harbor, or secrete, any such person under contract, or apprentice who has left the employment of employer or master, without the permission of such employer or master, the person or persons so offending shall be liable in damages to the employer or master, and shall, upon conviction, be punished by fine, in a sum not exceeding five hundred dollars, nor less than ten dollars, or by imprisonment in the county jail, or house of correction, for not more than six months, or by both such fine and imprisonment.

Sec. 2. Any person who shall employ any laborer or apprentice who is, at the time of such employment, under contract, for any period of time, to any other person, and before such time of service shall have elapsed, so as to deprive such first employer or the master of such apprentice, of the services of such laborer or apprentice, shall be deemed guilty of a misdemeanor, and, upon conviction thereof, before any Court of competent jurisdiction, shall be punished by a fine of not less than ten, nor more than five hundred dollars, for each and every offence, or by imprisonment in the county jail or house of correction, for a period not exceeding thirty days, or by both such fine and imprisonment, and shall be liable in damages to the party injured.

Sec. 3. Any person who shall discharge from his employment any laborer or apprentice, during the term of service agreed upon between such employer and such laborer or apprentice, or, at the expiration of such term of service, shall, upon the request of such laborer or apprentice, give to him or her a written certificate of discharge, and, upon refusal to do so, shall be deemed guilty of a misdemeanor, and, upon conviction, shall be punished by a fine not exceeding one hundred dollars.

Sec. 4. It shall be the duty of the Judges of the District Courts to give this Act specially in charge to the Grand Jury at each term of their respective Courts.

Approved November 1, 1866.

CHAPTER LXXXII
Source: University of North Texas: Gammel's Laws of Texas

CHAPTER LXXXII.

Sec. 1. What if I help a laborer or apprentice to leave employment of their employer or Master or Mistress?
1. You will be liable for damages to an employer, Master or Mistress if you encourage a laborer bound under contract or any bound apprentice to leave their employer, Master, or Mistress or feed, harbour, or hide the laborer or apprentice.
2. You will be fined between ten and five hundred dollars or imprisoned in the county jail or house of correction for up to six months.

Sec. 2. Can I employ a laborer or apprentice who is already employed under contract or bond?
1. If you employ a laborer or apprentice who is already employed under a contract or apprenticeship and the duration of their employment has not expired, you are guilty of a misdemeanor.
2. If convicted by a Court in the appropriate jurisdiction, you will be fined between ten and 500 dollars for each offence or imprisoned for up to thirty days in jail.
3. You will also be liable for all damages to the injured party.

Sec. 3. What procedures must I follow when I dismiss my apprentice or employer?
1. If you dismiss your laborer or apprentice from duties before the labor contract or at the end of the labor contract or apprenticeship, you must give the laborer or apprentice a written certificate of dismissal.
2. If you fail to give the laborer or apprentice a written certificate of dismissal, you will be guilty of a misdemeanor and fined up to one hundred dollars.

Chapter LXXXII in Plain English

APPENDIX II

Rhetorical Analysis of Texas Black Codes in Legalese and Plain English

In Appendix I of this book, I present the original legalese version of relevant sections of Texas Black Codes and the Plain English translation of each section. In this Appendix, I discuss the results of analysis of the Texas Black Codes (as evoking trust or distrust in rationale audiences) using the discourse markers from Table 2.1 of Chapter II. To translate the regulations from the traditional legalese style to Plain English, found in Appendix I, I used the criteria outlined in the Securities and Exchange Commission's "A Plain English Handbook: How to Create Clear SEC Disclosure Documents," which lists the following as common problems in disclosure documents: "long sentences, passive voice, weak verbs, superfluous words, legal and financial jargon, numerous terms, abstract words, unnecessary details, and unreadable design and layout" (Securities and Exchange Commission, 1998, p. 17)—"problems" I encountered as recently as 2001 when I worked as a regulation editor for State of Texas agencies. But given the drastically different political and social climate of the Texas Black Codes of 1866, would the removal of these stylistic choices alone, without the addition or removal of pertinent information, be enough to evoke trust?

This Appendix places these codes in their historical, political, and economic contexts and examines the costs and benefits of the original legalese version and my Plain English translation. As we read the original sections of the Texas Black Codes and my Plain English translations, we will attempt to answer the following questions: In Plain English translations of regulations, what is clarified, what is undone, and what is deferred? Would Plain English have made a difference in freed slaves' perceptions of Texas Black Codes? Is Plain English, as we define it today, as effective in evoking trust as we purport?

To rewrite the Texas Black Codes from their original text to Plain English, I used the question-and-answer format and addressed the "persons heretofore known as slaves" as "you." Today, this revision technique called the "you attitude," which Mike Markel describes as "looking at the situation from the reader's point of view and adjust content, structure, and tone to meet his or her needs" (Markel, 2006, pp. 340–341). While the "you attitude" is palatable today, in 1866 to promise "You will not be discriminated against" instead of "there shall be no discrimination against such persons" would be more than a Plain English revision but a gesture of respect that Texas legislators were, at the time, unwilling to extend to an African American audience. The revisions that you are about to read are more than differences in sentence structure, word choice, and tone, but some of the Plain English versions close a power distance between the Texas Legislature and black Texans that did not exist until nearly 100 years after the original text was written.

In Chapter CXXVIII, The Rights of "Persons of Color," the writers simultaneously expand and limit the rights of the recently freed slaves. It is important to note these rights as we move into discussions of contracting between laborers and landowners and the rights of the freed slaves in courts of law. In Chapter CXXVIII, Section 1, although this regulation, in legalese and Plain English, promises former slaves specific rights and liberties held by the majority of the state, in a report from Brigadier General and Assistant Commissioner E. M. Gregory to General O. O. Howard dated December 9, 1865, Gregory wrote, "In some portions of the State, especially it is the case where our troops have not been quartered, freedmen are restrained from their freedom and slavery as [?] virtually exists as the same as though the old system of oppression was still in force" (Gregory, 2002d, p. 69). Gregory's claim that blacks in Texas continued to work as slaves after the Emancipation Proclamation is common knowledge in Texas, where African Americans have celebrated Juneteenth (June 19), now a state holiday, since the receipt of the news of freedom in Galveston, Texas on June 19, 1865, two years after the Emancipation Proclamation was issued on January 1, 1863.

> On June 19 ("Juneteenth"), 1865, Union general Gordon Granger read the Emancipation Proclamation in Galveston, thus belatedly bringing about the freeing of 250,000 slaves in Texas. The tidings of freedom reached slaves gradually as individual plantation owners read the proclamation to their bondsmen over the months following the end of the war. The news elicited an array of personal celebrations, some of which have been described in *The Slave Narratives of Texas* (1974). The first broader celebrations of Juneteenth were used as political rallies and to teach freed African Americans about their voting rights. Within a short time, however, Juneteenth was marked by festivities throughout the state, some of which were organized by official Juneteenth committees.
>
> The day has been celebrated through formal thanksgiving ceremonies at which the hymn "Lift Every Voice" furnished the opening. In addition, public entertainment, picnics, and family reunions have often featured

dramatic readings, pageants, parades, barbecues, and ball games. Blues festivals have also shaped the Juneteenth remembrance. In Limestone County, celebrants gather for a three-day reunion organized by the Nineteenth of June Organization. Some of the early emancipation festivities were relegated by city authorities to a town's outskirts; in time, however, black groups collected funds to purchase tracts of land for their celebrations, including Juneteenth. A common name for these sites was Emancipation Park. In Houston, for instance, a deed for a ten-acre site was signed in 1872, and in Austin the Travis County Emancipation Celebration Association acquired land for its Emancipation Park in the early 1900s; the Juneteenth event was later moved to Rosewood Park. (Acosta, 2001, p. 1)

This yearly celebration, Juneteenth, is a remembrance not only of freedom but of slavery and the discriminatory laws that followed it. Interestingly enough, the last clause of Chapter CXXVIII, Section 1 states, "there shall be no discrimination against such persons [former slaves] in the administration of the criminal laws of this State," but Texas Black Codes were not criminal laws but mostly labor regulations. While the writer of Section 1 does list the new rights—"to make and enforce contracts, to sue and be sued, to inherit, purchase, lease, hold, sell, and convey real, personal and mixed estate; to make wills and testaments, and to have and enjoy the rights of personal security, liberty, and private property, and all remedies and proceedings for the protection and enforcement of the same" (11th Texas Legislature, 1866a, p. 1049), the Plain English and legalese versions of Chapter CXXVIII, Section 2 do little to inform blacks of the specifics of their newly acquired rights. For example, the writers of this regulation mention laws that "conflict with the provisions of this act," but do not specify the chapter or sections referenced. What laws conflict with this act? Is this information inadvertently or intentionally left out? While Michel Foucault saw currency in considering more than what is included in texts but also what and why certain information is excluded (Longo, 2000, p. 19), Jacques Derrida's notion of difference allows us to take note of more than what we see in text, but what is deferred (1982, p. 9). In this particular section of the Texas Black Codes, there is as much a reason to question the regulation about what is not written as there is for what is written.

With all of the technical information excluded from the Texas Black Codes, the Freedman's Bureau agents knew that the rights of freed slaves were often ignored and attempted to stand in the gap.

> The testimony of the Freedmen is admitted in the courts of some of the Judiciary Districts of this State, while in others it is not. It is my oppinion [sic] that their rights are not properly acknowledged and guarded by the Judiciary, but still there are indications that ere long they will receive that consideration to which they are untitled under the laws of the United States, and by the proclamation of the President. (Gregory, 2002d, pp. 67–68)

Chapter CXXVIII, Section 2 is our first example of overt discrimination in that it limits voting rights to white men and forbids interracial marriage. Even with these limitations, these two regulations are two of the most honest of the Texas Black Codes, in that the writers acknowledge race and the legal boundaries based on this construct. Texas Black Codes related to vagrancy laws, the apprenticeship of black children, and unfair labor contracts with black adults did not mention race. I will discuss the implications of this rhetorical maneuver in the rest of this Appendix.

In the Texas Black Codes that establish the penal code, Chapter LXXIII (11th Texas Legislature, 1866e), Section 1, Article 34; Article 39; and Article 408, we find discussions and definitions of race and ethnicity, specifically "persons of color" and Native Americans. While references to race are left out of the vagrancy, apprenticeship, and labor laws, we find clear definitions of race and ethnicity in these penal codes. Chapter LXXIII, Article 34 provides the terms "white persons" and "persons of color" to elucidate the distinction between these races. Still, neither term is referenced in any of the vagrancy, apprenticeship, or labor laws, which were enforced within these color lines and promulgated during this same legislative session that included these definitions of race. Article 34 demonstrates that there was no hesitance to include instructions for different races or ethnicities in regulations, but if this is the case, why were references to race left out of labor-related regulations (vagrancy, apprenticeship, and contract labor) that endorsed unfair labor contracts between blacks and whites? I include Chapter LXXIII, Section 1, Article 408, and its reference to "any Indian of wild or unfriendly tribes" to demonstrate that whites and blacks were not the only groups with instructions for the social and business interactions written into Texas law during the 11th Texas Legislative Session.

Chapter CXI (11th Texas Legislature, 1866b), Sections 1 through 10, represents Texas Black Codes that addressed the issue of criminalizing unemployed freed blacks. None of the Texas Black Codes in Chapter CXI pertaining to vagrancy fit into any of the trust categories, but all of these regulations were placed into various distrust categories for reasons I will outline here. The vagrancy regulations, although deceptive and vague, were some of the least harmful Texas Black Codes because there is little evidence of the enforcement of these regulations, while the apprenticeship and labor regulations discussed later were enforced and often voided by Freedman's Bureau agents (Crouch, 1999, p. 276). In Chapter CXI, Section 1, the original version of the regulation, which is written in a legalese style, makes no mention of race. The information left out of these sections, even after the Plain English revision, is the inclusion of a simple clause: "You are a vagrant if you are a recently freed slave who is unemployed." Thus, the Plain English translation does not change the deceptive nature of the regulation, which according to Barry Crouch, was used to "round up 'unemployed' blacks and force them into either private or public service" (1999, p. 265). This "round up" was certainly a means of forcing blacks into involuntary servitude. Crouch argued, "So called vagrants seem to have become a concern after the crops had been gathered and before the next seasonal cycle began" (p. 276). Thus, after laborers had completed field work outlined (and possibly agreed upon) in labor contracts, they were susceptible to involuntary labor during periods when field work was unavailable. While the first Section explains who can be assigned the title of "vagrant," the original legalese and Plain English translations of Section 2 assign power to certain officials to arrest and convict vagrants. Clearly, if a recently freed black Texan were to read or be read this regulation, there is certainly a possibility that the positions or job titles mentioned in the regulation would solicit feelings of distrust, because black Texans' relationships with courts and court officials were certainly not equal to that of their white peers. A Brenham, Texas agent wrote, "The operation of the vagrant law will depend much on the justice of the local tribunals . . . most likely to be abused to the oppression of the freedpeople for whom it was evidently intended" (Crouch, 1999, p. 276). Clearly, if a regulation mentions titles or positions of arbitrators that they cannot trust, the *ethos* of the agency promulgating the regulation is diminished.

Crouch wrote, "Because local and county officials complained that they had no funds to care for true black vagrants (those who had become so because of some specific action or catastrophe), or even the homeless, agents believed they had no recourse but to force these individuals to labor either for private employers or the public good" (1999, p. 276). In Chapter CXI, Section 3, it is clear that the Plain English version of this regulation does not negate the negative implications of regulating the labor of unemployed blacks, who could be arrested by private citizens who might be interested in having them work on their own land. There is no mention of any wages to be paid to a vagrant black Texan if brought before a judge or magistrate and made to work for a public or private citizen. There is certainly a motivation for white landowners who were previously slave owners to accuse and arrest blacks for vagrancy and bring them before the court. Thus, the inclusion of the private citizen in the regulation would certainly evoke distrust in the recently freed black Texan, even in the Plain English version.

In Chapter CXI, Section 4, the Plain English version of this regulation would be more helpful to an audience, in that jargon such as "proceed to ascertain, by evidence" can be replaced by "evaluate evidence" and superfluous words like "he shall be fined in any sum not more than ten dollars" can be replaced by "you can be fined as much as $10." Historian Barry Crouch notes the vagrancy law was ambiguous and therefore it was implemented and enforced inconsistently throughout the state. Crouch wrote, "Depending on the location of an agent, the vagrancy law did engender some ambiguity" (1999, p. 276). In this section, the ambiguity of the language used in the regulations promoted inconsistent enforcement and thus, would evoke distrust in rationale audiences who might witness inconsistent policy implementation in different parts of the state or even in the same area under different authorities (Aberbach & Walker, 1970,

p. 1199; Ting-Toomey, 1999, p. 223). Crouch also wrote, "Anthony M. Bryant of Sherman stated that, in his region, there was 'no attention whatever paid to the vagrant law,'" whereas "In Columbia [Texas] Duggan said that the law itself had not been applied, but he was 'compelled to threaten' two black men, who had abandoned their families, with its enforcement" (1999, p. 276). In the case of freed slaves who challenged their status as an apprentice because they were seeking employment, waiting for the next crop season, or even abandoning their families, their rights as accused are outlined in Chapter CXI. Section 5. The Plain English version of Section 5 attempts to clarify the rights of the accused. In the legalese version of the regulation, the main point is to advise the accuser that they can request a trial by jury. Unfortunately, this critical information is hidden in a nonessential clause. By subordinating "if he demand it," the author may very well be effective in hiding the right to a trial by jury from an uneducated audience. Here again, we find the recently freed slaves, though not referenced by position or race, would be required to interact with courts that did not acknowledge their testimony or concerns.

Chapter CXI, Section 6, even in its Plain English translation, is filled with abstract and inconsistent terms that violate guidelines for good technical communication. Both translations raise the following questions:

1. What "costs" does the regulation refer to?
2. In Section 4 of this same Chapter, the regulation writer states that fines for convicted vagrants will not exceed $10. Are these the same "fines and costs" mentioned in this Section that accumulate "at a rate of one dollar per day"? During this period, a fine accumulating at a rate of $1 per day seems excessive and would be impossible for an unemployed person to pay.
3. Can the words "costs" and "fines" be used interchangeably in this regulation? How do they differ?
4. Why has the term "officer" been introduced in this Section, while "justices," "courts," and "peace officer" were used in previous Sections?

In the Freedmen's Bureau policy circular dated October 17, 1865, Gregory wrote, "Freedmen committed as Vagrants may be set to work on roads or at any other labor by the Authorities which provide their Support or they may be turned over to an Agent of this Bureau" (2002e, p. 21). In its historical context, this section suggests that a convicted vagrant will be put to work on city roads with some "Support" during times when their labor is not needed in the fields. Although the Freedmen's Bureau regulation makes provision for their input regarding the labor from the Freedmen's Bureau, there is no mention of the Freedmen's Bureau in the Texas Black Codes. Barry Crouch suggests that local courts implemented their own regulations regarding vagrants without input from the Freedmen's Bureau.

In Chapter CXI, Section 7, mislabeled as Section 8, Crouch provides evidence that the regulation was not enforced. The inclusion of the word "may" in Section 7 allows for flexibility or inconsistency in the enforcement of this regulation, and the fact that a "credible person" is given the authority to issue a warrant for the arrest of a vagrant makes the regulation ambiguous. How is "credible person" defined? Neither the Plain English nor legalese versions of the regulation provide a definition of this abstract term. It is likely that a "credible person" as defined by the enforcers of this regulation would not be viewed as "credible" by the freedmen, especially if white landowners were included in this definition. Thus, the terms "may" and "credible person" certainly allow for inconsistency between the regulation and its actual enforcement. Although the Texas Black Codes regarding vagrancy were not often enforced, there is evidence that local authorities did follow Chapter CXI, Section 7, about which Barry Crouch argues "The vagrancy part of the 1866 Texas Black Codes were used sparingly against black Texans; more often, local laws were implemented" (1999, p. 276). Although I do not have examples of these local laws, it is clear that both the legalese and Plain English versions of any implementation of this Texas Black Code would have the same result on the freed people—unemployed black people were legally obligated to work for free. Fortunately, it does not appear that vagrancy codes had the negative impact of other apprenticeship laws, which are referenced in Chapter CXI, Section 9. There is ambiguity in both the legalese and Plain English versions of Section 9. There is no mention of the fact that "apprentices," under the Texas Black Codes are black children and no Chapter or Section number is referenced to identify the "Criminal Code in relation to the same offences." What will occur if the "fines and penalties prescribed in this Act" do not conform to the provisions in the criminal code? Important information is missing from both versions of the regulation. Now, we will examine the harshest of the Texas Black Codes, the apprenticeship laws.

In a letter from E. M. Gregory to O. O. Howard dated April 18, 1866, Gregory wrote,

> The schools for Freedmen are reported satisfactory and flourishing. . . .They report a total attendance of Forty-Five hundred and Ninety Scholars of whom Twenty-eight hundred and thirty are children, and Seventeen hundred and sixty adult. . . .Though we are compeled [sic] to meet, in the inception of our work, all the prejudices and hostilities incident to Such an effort in our community, while every shade of opposition short of actual violence was used against our teachers, zeal in no instance [illegible word; looks like "proved"] been yielded [??], or a school once organized been suffered to be dispersed terrorized or broken up. (2002a, pp. 194–195)

Months later, in a report to Freedmen's Bureau Lieutenant J. P. Richardson dated January 31, 1867, James T. Butler responded to a question on his monthly report regarding education and recently freed slaves. Butler wrote,

> There are in Huntsville about two-hundred colored children between the ages of seven and eighteen, who could and should attend school. Knowing this fact last summer and expecting that the Bureau would apist [sic] in paying a teacher so as to make the tuition comparatively nothing, thereby enabling all parents to send all their children to school." (2003, p. 6)

Gregory and Butler's words imply that the Federal Government made provisions to send black children to school, while the Texas Black Codes made plans and laws for these same children to be apprenticed as laborers, often without wages or the consent of their parents.

In Chapter LXIII (11th Texas Legislature, 1866f), Sections 1 through 11, I examine the most harmful Texas Black Codes, which make obvious the effects on the population of freed blacks of their exclusion from participation as jurors and citizens with equal rights. The apprenticeship of black minors with little regard for the voices of their parents, families, and guardians and the latitude afforded to white "masters" and "mistresses" coupled with the rhetorical strategies that hide the definitions of terms and extent of punishments provides evidence that the legalese style can contribute to a language of distrust.

In Chapter LXIII, Section 1, Crouch's definition of black orphans makes the intent of this section of the code much more threatening than if received without the knowledge of the plight of black minors whose parents had been sold to neighboring states and thus could not consent or disallow the apprenticeship of their children to white landowners.

> The usual consensus of the courts, generally manned by former Confederates, was that orphaned black children were better off if they were bound to white families. They quickly shunted aside black objections to this practice and indentured the children to service for a decade or more. . . . Slavery was responsible for the aberrant definition in the postwar era. With parents being sold away to other states and communication nonexistent or sporadic, the whereabouts of parents was often lost in memory. (Crouch, 1999, p. 268)

The regulation makes provision for blacks in the community who were willing to care for the minors in the absence of their parents. Although there is no definition for guardian, the regulation seems harmless when reading it outside of the realm of its social and political contexts.

According to Crouch, those persons who were responsible for enforcing apprenticeships obviously misused their power, especially when enforcing regulations on recently freed slaves. Thus, black parents, guardians, and minors reading or being read apprenticeship codes were informed that their rights and protections were in the hands of the very people who terrorized federal Freedmen's Bureau agents in the streets.

In the report to Freedmen's Bureau Lieutenant J. P. Richardson dated January 31, 1867, James T. Butler responded to a question on his monthly report regarding criminal offenses in his jurisdiction. Butler wrote, "An unprovoked apsault [sic] with intent to murder. The complainant was haping [sic] along the Public Square of Huntsville, when Burgess, in broad daylight ipsued [sic] out of the store, presented a derringer, loaded, cocked at complainants heart, and bid him, 'if he had anything to say, to say it quick, for in one minute he was to be a dead man.'" Butler identified himself as the complainant and Burgess as the county sheriff. Later in the report as a suggestion to Freedmen's Bureau officials, Butler wrote, "The only difficulties I labor under in the world, and which could be very easily remedied, is a set of contemptibly [sic] disloyal civil officers. They are continually annoying and haraping [sic] me, which makes my duties a burden, and since the promulgation of General Hancock's orders, they have become so elated with the idea of "Texas civil law" that they boldy defy the Government and its officers; the planters [landowners] when ordered in to effect settlements positively refuse to come, and say that everything is turner [sic] over to the civil authorities now, and I have no jurisdiction. (Butler, 1867, pp. 1–12)

In both the Plain English and original version of Section 2, terms such as "competent person" and "suitable" are not defined and give the County Judge a lot of room for interpretation. Criteria defining a competent and suitable master or mistress must be defined as well as "all minors whose parent or parents have not means." How poor must a family be to have their children apprenticed? This language gave those in power the ability to apprentice black minors based on vague and inconsistent criteria. In Chapter LXIII, Section 3, there is no mention of the parties involved in the agreement that should be approved by the County Judge. There is no mention of the minor's father, mother, guardian or even the minors over age 14 who can agree to apprenticeship. What if conflicts arise between the minor's parents and the master or mistress? The fact that mention of these parties is missing provides grounds for Gregory's claim that some courts did not admit the testimony of freed slaves, and their rights under the law were very limited. In the Freedmen's Bureau report dated December 9, 1865, Gregory suggests that county courts were not always open to testimony or records presented by blacks (2002d, pp. 67–68). Thus, if the age of the minors were in question, testimony regarding a minor's age by parents, guardians, or other black relatives may not be accepted in court.

The intent and language used in Chapter LXIII, Section 4 is certainly inconsistent with its application. Again, without the historical contexts, the Plain English and legalese versions of the regulations appear to be less harmful or fair. In both versions of the regulation, "court testimony" is very likely to be limited to testimony by nonblacks who would have little interests in proving a minor to be older than 14, the age that a minor can legally decide not to be apprenticed. Chapter LXIII, Section 5 contains abstract terms like "sufficient," "humanely," and "faithful" giving the "masters," "mistresses," and county judges leeway in meeting the requirements in the regulation. Although the regulation does not allow parents or guardians of apprentices to decide how they would spend monies recovered from successful lawsuits against masters and mistresses, the regulation is one of the only Texas Black Codes written to protect the black laborer. More importantly, the regulation alerts the master and mistress of the possibility of financial loss if they do not meet the terms of the bond.

Notice in Chapter LXIII, Section 6, the word "power" is used to describe the master and mistress' right to physically punish a black child. Again, an abstract term such as "moderate" allows the master or mistress a lot of room for interpretation. As early as Plato's *The Laws*, the philosopher argued, "But you ought not to use the word 'moderate' in the way you did just now, you must say what 'moderate' means and how big or small it may be. If you don't you must realize that a remark such as you made still has some way to go before it can be law" (1970, p. 181). Also in Section 6, "as may be necessary and proper" is subjective and allows for inconsistent enforcement and implementation of the regulation. Clearly vagueness of terms could be used to make legitimate the physical abuse of minors as shown in Crouch's statement,

> One agent in Sterling encountered a youngster, previously apprenticed by the county court, who had obviously received "harsh treatment." The Bureau agent believed that the young man (no age given) was old enough to work for more than provisions and clothes and should be compensated for his labor. The Bureau agent refused to release the boy to the planter until the contract was signed, with the agent as the guardian, which entitled the minor to earnings. (Crouch, 1999, p. 271)

The fact that the employer is allowed to physically harm the employee delegates the employee to a place less than equal to the employer, not only in terms of employment but also in terms of their positions in society. In both the original and Plain English versions of Chapter LXIII, Section 7, the master and mistress are given permission to recapture a black minor who leaves employment—Plain English does not erase these permissions. Although Section 7 makes provision for the apprentice to be freed from indentured servitude if the court finds good reason, there is provision for the apprentice to be punished for leaving. This is clearly a sign of forced or involuntary labor.

In Chapter LXIII, Section 8, phrases like, "That in case any master or mistress of any apprentice may desire," "shall have the privilege," and "released from liability," indicate that the master and mistress were certainly afforded more rights and respect than the apprentices in terminating apprenticeships. There is no equitable regulation that would allow an apprentice to decide to end an apprenticeship, except after a master or mistress has already violated the bond. In Section 9, the first few words of the legalese version of this code seem to address illegal actions of apprentices: "It shall not be legal for any apprentice . . ." but this code is actually written to inform the master and mistress that it is illegal for them to take the apprentice, whose subject position in this regulation is expressed in terms of an object, not an employee with rights. The potential lawbreaker, the master or mistress, is not mentioned until the end of the regulation. Finally, the Plain English translation, which addresses the master or mistress, is effective in highlighting the responsibilities of the master and mistress and their role as potential lawbreakers. Although this section addresses the obligations of the mistress and master, Section 10 is unique in that the legalese and Plain English versions speak directly to the apprentice and his or her rights. This regulation outlines those circumstances where the apprentice is free to make a decision to leave or stay with the master or mistress. The fact that the black audience and their rights are addressed in the same code, without the use of passive voice hiding the subject is unique in this set of regulations. Also, the statement, "at the pleasure of said apprentice" is unusual in that it assigns the apprentice some decision-making power and respect. Still, no fines, costs, or imprisonment is assigned to the master or mistress for failing to consult the Court before taking the apprentice out of court for more than 30 days.

In "To Enslave the Rising Generation: The Freedmen's Bureau and the Texas Black Code," Barry A. Crouch wrote, "Texas blacks endeavored to take care of their own and bring orphaned or so-called "parentless" children into the confines of the black community" (1999, p. 268). In Chapter LXIII, Section 11, a guardian or relative attempting to provide shelter for the minor black child is criminalized and the minor is treated as property. Words in both the Plain English and legalese versions of the regulations such as "harbor," "conceal" and "entice away" evoke images of a runaway slave, not a contracting employee, and certainly not a free child. Fines are mentioned as punishment for those attempting to help these minors. One field officer, Gary Barrett, wrote, "as it only requires a notification in the papers of the intention to indenture, and as very few freed people can read, those interested immediately have not knowledge of the apprenticeship until after its consummation by the Court" (Crouch, 1999, p. 273). In Section 12, there is ambiguity in the Plain English and legalese versions of this regulation. Who is responsible for posting the notice? Why is permission needed from guardians and not parents? (Parents are mentioned in Section 2 of Chapter LXIII.) Gary Barrett argues that the notices of intention to indenture were not read by the black guardians or parents with the power to attest the apprenticeship (Crouch, 1999, p. 273). Most importantly, if the recently freed slaves could read the regulation, the public notice information, which is vital for parents and guardians wishing to attest the apprenticeship, is not mentioned until the second portion of the regulation.

Contractual theory, which is fundamentally an assertion that "a promise is legally enforceable if it is given as part of a bargain and it is unenforceable otherwise" is clearly negated in many of the following labor regulations that are written to negotiate the labor of recently freed black adults (Cooter & Ulen, 1988, p. 214). In the following analyses, note that many of the regulations that would evoke distrust in postbellum African American audiences would endorse contracts that are void of bargain or participation by the freed slaves. In the circular dated October 17, 1865, Gregory wrote, "I. All contracts with Freedmen for labor for the period of one Month and upwards must be conside [?] to writing, Approved by an Agent of this Bureau and one Copy deposited with him in proper case he shall require security" (Gregory, 2002e, p. 20), while Chapter LXXX (11th Texas Legislature, 1866d), Section 1 of the Texas Black Codes designates local officials and "disinterested persons" as witnesses and processors of the contact and agreement. In the report to Lieutenant J. P. Richardson dated January 31, 1867, James T. Butler wrote, "Today a contract was brought to my notice, which the employer forced the freedpeople to sign. I disapproved the contract and informed the employer and the freedpeople" (Butler, 1867, p. 7). Butler's Freedmen's Bureau report provides evidence that landowners forced some freed persons to sign these contracts and that some contract negotiations were not followed as outlined by Texas Black Codes and certainly not as outlined by Freedmen's Bureau regulations, which required the contracting parties bring their contracts before Freedmen's Bureau staff for approval.

In Chapter LXXX, Section 1, both the Plain English versions of this regulation raise as many questions as answers. Who will write the contract? Who is required to read the contract to the laborer? Clearly, the legalese version of the regulation makes these questions less obvious by hiding the lack of an actor in passive voice. Much of the Plain English version is also written in passive voice because the original regulation does not designate a person to write or read the contract. Again, the fact that most of the laborers were "persons of color" is also left out of this regulation. In the letter from Gregory to Howard dated January 31, 1866, Gregory wrote, "The blacks were willing to work asking only that the promises made them by the planters be enforced by the Government. Under these conditions contracts were made freely with the freedmen and approved by the Bureau on liberal terms. There is a great variety of contracts between them and their employers and much vagueness of terms" (Gregory, 2002b, p. 122). This vagueness was certainly preceded by the vague terms laid out in the Texas Black Codes. In both the legalese and Plain English of Chapter LXXX, Section 2, terms such as "harsh treatment" or "cause" are certainly too abstract or subjective for black laborers to depend on when deciding to leave an employer. Still, this regulation does lay out the terms of agreement that would likely be acceptable to anyone interested in agreeing to a voluntary labor contract. In both styles, the regulation appears to be fair in that it allows the laborer to choose an employer, leave if there is good cause, and lose wages if the laborer leaves without good cause. It outlines terms of an agreement that would likely be enforceable even today. Most importantly, there are not excessive fines, confinement, or physical punishment for leaving the employment. This language recommends a more positive relationship between whites and recently freed slaves and would probably evoke trust.

In Section 3, the Texas Black Code writers quickly revert to the strategy of hiding the actor. Who is depositing the contract with the County Clerk? It is unlikely that the laborer wrote the contract or "deposited" it with the County Clerk, so the use of passive voice is effective in hiding the agent in this regulation. In cases when the agent is hidden, Plain English forces the disclosure of this information. While the Plain English version of Section 3 makes the reader, who is either the laborer or the employer, the actor. The language in the Plain English and legalese version of Chapter LXXX, Section 4 makes no distinctions between laborers and employers. In Section 4, black laborers and white landowners are treated equally, charged equal amounts of money, and there are no signs, even in the historical record, of discrimination in the enforcement of this particular regulation. In Section 5, instead of hiding or removing information, the writer adds nine words that would make an enormous difference to a black child in 1866. In Section 5, the writer uses almost identical language as the Freedmen's Bureau Code 33.II, For Plantation Labor, but Black Code writers added, "shall be binding on all minors of said families." Basically, the additional language would require minors to work. The Freedmen's Bureau code states that the contract would embrace all members of the family, whereas the Texas Black Codes states that it would embrace the labor of all members of the family. This section of the Black Codes, in legalese and Plain English, would evoke distrust in blacks because it is deceptive. The federal regulation, which this code was supposed to be modeled after, did not state that minors were required to work. The Freedmen's Bureau intended to provide schools for recently freed minors, not require minors to work, as they would have under the slave system.

In contrast to the contradictions in the intent of the Federal Government and State Government explained in the previous section, Chapter LXXX, Section 6 appears to be in line with the intentions of the Freedmen's Bureau regulation 33.II, For Plantation Labor. In the circular dated October 17, 1865, Gregory wrote,

> Such contracts will be a lien upon the Crop of which not more than one half will [be] removed untill [sic] all payments have been made, and untill [sic] the contract shall have been released by an Agent of this Bureau or Justice of the Peace in case it is impractable [sic] to procure the Services of Such Agents. (2002e, p. 20)

Also, in the letter from Gregory to Howard dated January 31, 1866, Gregory wrote, "In many instances, instead of wages, a portion of the crop ranging from 1/4 to 1/2 according to the special conditions of each case is pledged to the laborers and the instances are not infrequent in addition to high percentage of the expected crop, the planter boards and lodges his workmen gratis" (2002b, p. 123).

The legalese and Plain English versions fail to stipulate who is restricted from removing crops from the plantation before wages are paid, owners or laborers. Again, the person taking action is not clearly defined. This style of writing promotes ambiguity and allows for inconsistent implementation and enforcement of the regulation. Thus, the use of "You" in a regulation is not effective unless it is used throughout the entire regulation and passive voice is consistently avoided. Chapter LXXX, Section 7, of the Texas Black Codes could also be viewed as one that would evoke trust in black laborers had the word "willfully" not been included as a caveat that could certainly be used in the employee's favor. An easy argument for the employer is that they did not "willfully" violate the contract. There is no equal disclaimer in Texas Black Codes regulating the duties and responsibilities of laborers. There is no mention of whether or not they "willfully" injure animals; there are only penalties. Here, the white employees certainly receive favorable treatment and a clear way out of fines and penalties. In the letter to Benjamin G. Harris Esq. and Foreman of the Grand Jury of Panola County Texas dated January 20, 1866, Gregory stated, "Many of the freedmen were last year defrauded of their earnings. . . . Better treatment and prompt pay will correct this distrust sooner than a Brigade of 'Provost Marshals'" (2002c, p. 112). Chapter LXXX, Section 8 of the Texas Black Codes arms the landowners and local officials with the authority needed to deduct wages from black laborers. Although Section 8 states that the employer should provide medical care for the laborer and continue compensation until the laborer recovers from illness, the Texas Black Code provides stipulations for punishing a laborer who states that he is ill. Both the Plain English and legalese versions of the regulation fail to answer the following questions:

1. Who will report the laborer to the Justice of the Peace or Mayor?
2. Who will force the laborer to work on roads?
3. How will the employer determine if the illness is "feigned"?

Clearly, this section attacks the laborers work ethic, a challenge further cemented in postbellum popular culture in "coon songs" and dehumanizing cartoons where the black laborer was shiftless and lazy and would "feign" illness (Dorman, 1988, pp. 450–471). In reality (and understandably so) black Texas laborers did not work as hard as they did during slavery as expressed in the September 21, 1865 letter from Gregory to Benjamin Harris: "The general report of Planters and employers is that the freedmen are not doing as much as under the slave system and yet the crops will be saved [?] to the country" (2002f, pp. 109–113).

Chapter LXXX, Section 9, of the Texas Black Code, in both styles of writing, suggests that if a laborer is ill for more than 3 days, they are in jeopardy of being reported to local authorities and facing punishment. This is clearly excessive punishment that is not faced by employers who fail to meet their contractual obligations. Surprisingly, most of the information in the legalese version of this regulation is relatively clear and written in active voice. Finally, a vague term such as "disobedience" is defined within the same section that it is first used; this is an obvious attempt at clarity. With all of the demands of the employer on the laborer, brevity and sincerity are goals of the writer; this is the longest and arguably the harshest of the Texas Black Codes. In the Plain English version, I attempted to reorganize the regulation so that the reader could decipher the requirements of the laborer from the rights of the employer. By separating the duties and requirements of the laborer from the rights of the employer, it is easy to see that this regulation is written from the employer's viewpoint and with the employer's rights in mind. The excessive fines and duties, including the fact that laborers are said to be off on Sundays but clearly are not, is consistent with Gregory's report that in many instances, contract labor was no different than slavery. Again, in Chapter LXXX, Section 10, when the Texas Black Code writers attempted to transfer information about the duties and requirements of laborers, they seem to communicate in a clear style of writing and use active voice. The first word identifies the audience. My Plain English version of the regulation is very similar to the legalese version, but I do include subsections for sake of clarity. Also, the Texas Black Code writer used the phrase "the class of laborers" to differentiate this group from other citizens and requiring them to be "especially polite to their employer, his family and guests." There is not an equivalent admonition in the Texas Black Codes protecting the rights of laborers, only the requirement that apprentices are treated humanely in Chapter LXIII (11th Texas Legislature, 1866f, pp. 979–981). As in the previous regulation, the claims that laborers had Sundays and night hours off are fallacies that are quickly clarified by the suggestion that employers and their families could call on laborers anytime they really needed their services.

Clearly, the strict labor requirements mandated in the adult labor laws within the Texas Black Codes did not always appear to contradict federal policy, as evidenced and communicated in Gregory's October 17, 1865, policy circular:

> IV. But as Many persons have not learned the binding force of a contract and that "freedom" does not mean "living with labor," it is further ordered that when any employer under this Order shall make oath before a Justice of the Peace acting as Agent of this Bureau and having local jurisdiction that one of his employees has been absent from his employ for a longer period than one day without just cause, or for an aggregate term of more than 5 days in one Month the Authorities shall proceed against such person as a Vagrant. (2002e, p. 21)

The major difference between the Texas Black Codes and federal policy is that Freedmen's Bureau agents wanted the labor and vagrancy laws applied fair and across color lines. In his January 20, 1866, letter to Benjamin G. Harris, Gregory instructed, "Apply the Vagrant and criminal laws of the state to Black and White alike, and meet [sic] out to each offender the stern discipline of [sic] justice" (2002c, p. 111).

Finally, in Chapter LXXX, Section 11, terms of dismissal appear to be fair, but the distribution of power of those persons responsible for hearing the laborer's appeal is not clear. Will the citizen selected by the laborer have the same power as the citizen selected by the employer? What is the relationship or decision-making power of the two citizens to the Justice of the Peace? Are laborers, if "persons of color," considered citizens of the county?

While contemporary regulations provide help for children and laborers who work in abusive or unhealthy environments, the following regulations vow to punish those attempting to help the freed blacks and their children. In Chapter LXXXII (11th Texas Legislature, 1866c), Sections 1 through 3, we find regulations that suggest that those attempting to help freed blacks to leave these environments, which white landowners and members of the 11th Texas Legislature deemed suitable, should face some of the worst punishments and fines in the Texas Black Codes. It is ironic that during this period in history, these persons attempting to help freed blacks who found themselves back in physically abusive and slave-like work situations would be punished instead of lauded as public servants.

Barry A. Crouch (1999) wrote "Texas blacks endeavored to take care of their own and bring orphaned or so-called 'parentless' children into the confines of the black community" (p. 268). Chapter LXXXII, Section 1, is the second example of a Texas Black Code that threatens persons attempting to help apprentices and black laborers leave their employers. This particular regulation records the harshest fines and prison terms of the Texas Black Codes. Why is there a need for such harsh penalties against persons attempting to help apprentices and laborers leave employment? Why are the fines and punishments for persons "enticing" apprentices and laborers more stringent than even those enforced against laborers? The historical record asserts that there were blacks who attempted to help slaves escape, and there is certainly the possibility that if labor contracts were enforced as if the slave system was still in effect, there was still the need for laborers and apprentices to escape their employees. The words "entice" and "persuade" in lieu of "escape" or "run away," suggests employment of laborers and apprentices was not a negative experience. The only persons operating outside of the law were those enticing and persuading the laborers and apprentices to leave "good" jobs. The Section 2 writer is attempting to dissuade those attempting to employ black laborers and apprentices already under contract with other employers. With such harsh punishments and fines, there is little incentive for other employers to offer competitive wages to laborers and apprentices and little incentive to help those who are being treated unfairly a means of escape. Both the legalese and Plain English versions of the regulation would likely evoke distrust in recently freed slaves because their ability to engage in free market activities, like other laborers, are limited by such regulations.

In translating Chapter LXXXII, Section 3 from legalese to Plain English, I had difficulty placing the phrase "upon the request of such laborer or apprentice" within the context of the regulation. What request of the laborer or apprentice is the employer making? Is the employer requesting permission to release the laborer or apprentice earlier than the term of the contract or apprenticeship or even at the end of the agreed-upon time? If so, this information needs to be clearly spelled out. Still, finally, the laborer and apprentice are protected under the law and allowed written verification of their release for service. This is one of the few sections that would likely evoke trust in recently freed slaves.

DISCOURSE ANALYSIS OF TEXAS BLACK CODES IN LEGALESE AND PLAIN ENGLISH

In my translation of Texas Black Codes to Plain English in Appendix I, it is easy to see how Plain English regulations, without consideration of the historical context of the regulation and its audience, can remain vague, and legalese—for all practical purposes, anyway—even less clear. After translating all of the Texas Black Codes from legalese to Plain English in Appendix I, my decision to classify many of the Texas Black Codes sections as evoking trust and distrust had as much to do with intent and content of the regulations, as viewed in the historical contexts, as with the style of the regulations. Before I translated the Texas Black Codes from legalese to Plain English, I anticipated that some of the distrust categories would become irrelevant in the Plain English translations. I thought, "Language used in the regulations is inconsistent with actions in the enforcement of the regulations or intent of the regulations" with a precise application of the Plain English style would force the writer to be, if nothing else, honest (Aberbach & Walker, 1970, p. 1199; Ting-Toomey, 1999, p. 223). But in these translations from legalese to Plain English, especially in cases where making language more honest makes it more sinister, it is obvious that it takes more than short sentences and familiar words to make language plain. The plain style requires honesty that is manifested not by short words or sentences but by even more detail and possibly an even more exhaustive consideration of context than legalese. Plain English, especially when using "You," requires the writer to consider the audience and speak to them. In Texas Black Codes, where the writers employed what Crouch called a "nondiscriminatory façade that fooled no one" (1999, p. 264), the writers were not required to address their black audience, were not required to be honest with this audience, and were in turn free to write without consideration of the emotional, logical, and distrustful responses of a rationale audience.

APPENDIX III

Contextual Inquiry Transcript

WHY DO YOU WRITE REGULATIONS?

Policy Writer A: "Administrative rules come from within the agency. We are much clearer now about how regulations are different from policy and procedure. We understand that we can't require the provider to do anything that isn't in the rule. We understand that we can't put things in policy [standards] without it being in the rule [regulation]. The daycare standards are now cross-referenced in the regulation. The standard is now the rule. In daycare we consolidated standards to replace duplication. Half of each set of regulations was duplicated in each set of standards, so to increase consistency, we realized that it doesn't matter what type of facility the kids are in; there are still certain expectations about what good out-of-home care is."

Policy Writer B: "Most rule changes are suggested from within the agency. It depends on if another agency is also looking at this problem. We sometimes have to change rules as a result of another division with the department. It could be a recurring issue from the field, staff, or providers."

Policy Writer C: "Rules are changed as a result of changes in law. We are currently changing standard numbers to make sure that standards refer providers to rules and laws. The whole idea of consolidating 11 steps of standards into 3 sets of standards is difficult to understand. It's [consolidation] the way that state agencies are going in trying to make things better. I hope that they get to the point in residential standards that daycare standards has. There are some standards and types of facilities that are totally different and require different safeguards."

HOW DO YOU WRITE REGULATIONS?

Policy Writer A: "There is no training for a subject-matter expert, and this makes it difficult for a new person to get onboard. Working in teams and asking questions helps. I had the assumption that the question-and-answer [Plain

English] format would increase the number of rules. We found out a year after the Plain English minimum standards were approved that the rules still need to be clarified. We had the same problems with staff and providers regarding the regulations. We found out the hard way that Plain English doesn't negate the need for more training. The need to clarify and the inability for field staff to make judgments is still a problem in Plain English."

Policy Writer B: "We don't write rules as much as we would like to. We're rewriting all of the standards. In the revision, we are getting rid of all clarification memos because they've been enforced as if they were rules, but they aren't. Some need to be in rule; it's a long-term goal. We now have to go through HHSC, which is a complicated process before it [proposed rule] goes to Council. The Council doesn't have the authority to make changes or decisions. The benefit to consolidating is consistency; when you have too many sets of standards it's difficult. Originally, I set up a draft with the core standards and then the breakouts, additional standards that apply to unique groups. Washington State also has a question-and-answer format. No matter what kind of rule you write, there are always all types of problems that pop up that you don't expect. We've had several focus groups and work groups with providers, and now the rules are clear, but it doesn't leave room for interpretation. They can't have it both ways, clarity and objectivity."

Policy Writer C: "Rulewriting is collaborative. We have to work together as a group to make sure that things in standards and regulations are the same. We also have to work with CPS and legal. We have to work with the automation staff to see how the regulation change will impact Class, the automation system for division. We make sure that Policy Clarifications are in rule. How-to-complys must be in rule. Texas is innovative, and although we object to some of the changes, the product that will come out of the consolidations and Plain English will be a model and cutting edge. All of the other groups are looking for copies of our daycare standards. Some providers and staff look at the question-and-answer format as too prescriptive and don't believe it gives them room to make judgments. Legalese left more room for field staff and providers to be subjective. Providers used legalese against the agency because of the wiggle room. In this agency, unlike other agencies, attorneys don't write the rules; subject-matter experts do. So, you learn by examples from your coworkers, working together as a group. You learn a lot just from doing it. There was a legal attorney that was close to the program to answer questions but no longer."

WHO IS THE AUTHOR?

Policy Writer A: "Standards are to protect children. Administrative rules are to protect the providers. We use administrative rules when providers are new or in trouble. I learned the hard way that the final rule doesn't look like what I wrote. New rule writers need to understand that they don't own the rule, and they need to understand that it's not theirs anymore. I learned to write the best rule I can before everyone else gets involved. Once I think it's my draft, it's over. I understand the public process, but it's painful to see the rule changes. Knowledge bases are lost when staff changes."

Policy Writer B: "Rules are often changed regardless of the fact that the writers have research to support the draft as it was originally written."

Policy Writer C: "We will totally lose ownership once the legislators review rules. One constituent can call a legislator and change the law. As the gatekeeper, we have knowledge base that the legislators don't have, especially based on the comment of one angry provider. People in agencies leave, and bring in experiences, and things changed based on a person, even if they don't have the knowledge base."

DESCRIBE YOUR REVISION PROCESS

Policy Writer A: "I received over 16,000 comments on the daycare rules; all Child Care Licensing staff in State Office [Austin] helped me to make the responses. The more layers of review, the less time we have to respond to comments. By no longer having a board, providers can no longer make oral comments in the board meetings; this circumvents a piece of the public comment process. The new council provides as much testimony as we might have heard from the public because the council can be opinionated about things that are not perceived to most as a big deal."

Policy Writer B: "Each time we've gotten a new administrator, we can try to defend the rule, but if it's one person making the final decision. There is really no way to present the research that you have for leaving the room as it is."

Policy Writer C: "The Council has been demoted from a Board, and it's not clear what power they will have to revise rules." [At this point, one of the agency attorneys entered the crypt and began a conversation with Policy Writer A about daycare policy. Policy Writer A spoke with the attorney for about 10 minutes regarding the interpretation of a Child Care Licensing policy before we continued our discussion about the regulatory writing. Policy Writer B later informed me that this attorney has a natural talent for writing Plain English regulations that other policy writers and attorneys struggle with.]

DO YOU COLLABORATE WITH OTHER ORGANIZATIONS AND RESOURCES WHEN WRITING REGULATIONS?

Policy Writer A: "Part of my research is usually from other nationally recognized programs, Child Welfare League. We look at what other states are doing. Try to see what's going on, although with daycare, the administrators told us, "We are Texas" and no one really cared what was going on in other states. During the last legislative session, legislators passed a law for duplicating regulations with the health department because the standards and requirements can say that some health standards are covered by another agency. Duplication of rules in immunizations is what could be considered. CCL cross-referenced the health department regulations in our rules; it's not ideal as far as customer service, but conflicts have been removed."

Policy Writer B: "NARA has information for finding information about other states' daycare rules, but residential childcare doesn't have an equivalent. Sometimes these regulations are in different agencies than the childcare regulations; this makes it difficult to find out how to find residential regulations from other states."

Policy Writer C: "We can go into a national research table to show what the national consensus is on the rule. Stakeholders have more chances to influence the process than before. A lot of the other states have departments that are under the same umbrella and that may make it easier to work with other divisions like TWC, et cetera. Now they get into a situation where they do things that impact TWC, health department, fire department, and vice versa. There is little coordination between these agencies. Each agency has their own goals and directives, and they are never contacted by the fire department."

MEETINGS WITH INDIVIDUAL POLICY WRITERS IN THEIR WRITING ENVIRONMENTS: QUESTIONS ABOUT AUDIENCE

1. Who will read these regulations? (Attorneys? Daycare Owners? Daycare Directors? Who else?)

Policy Writer A: "Regulations are written for licensing staff and providers. Providers are priority."

Policy Writer C: "Licensing representatives [field investigators], providers, and Child Protective Services. CPS owns a child-placing agency and monitors their foster homes."

2. Do you know the demographic makeup of the people who will read these regulations?

Policy Writer A: "Reflective of Texas. The ethnicity is probably similar to the national average. Females, average age around 36, high school diploma. Department of Labor has stats online."

Policy Writer B: "Mostly white males and females, maybe?"

Policy Writer C: "What I write affects minorities. I write regulations for criminal background checks of providers, and this disproportionately affects minorities."

3. Does the ethnic makeup of your audience affect the language you use in your regulations?

Policy Writer A: "Vietnamese population is increasing in the Houston and Arlington areas; may be of concern."

Policy Writer B: "The main thing is that the rules are clear and of the best interests of the children."

Policy Writer C: "The system is lacking because we don't consider that minority families have different family practices."

4. Do you know the educational backgrounds of the people who read your regulations?

Policy Writer A: "I write for an eighth-grade level. I have used Microsoft Word's readability scale for daycare regulations."

Policy Writer B: "Most administrators have to have a degree and pass a licensing exam." [This policy writer writes regulations that are directed at degreed administrators certified to run a specific type of residential facility, not daycare owners.]

Policy Writer C: "There are more educated providers in residential centers than daycare centers. Residential facility owners are required to have at least a GED or high school diploma. A lot of registered family homeowners, including many Hispanics, can't read. We have to remember whom we're writing for."

5. Which writing style does your audience prefer? And why?

Policy Writer A: "I thought that Plain English would be easier, but I still get questions from field staff about what things mean. For example, rules that mention things that a provider may need like, 'self-closing, self-locking gates' is very unclear to many. We have to do a lot of interpreting with Plain English."

Policy Writer C: "Providers don't understand legalese and don't apply it. They do read the Plain English. Providers have complained that the new rules are too clear, "yes" or "no." They wanted us to write descriptive answers in the question and answer format, not yes or no."

QUESTION ABOUT TRUST

Are you concerned with writing regulations that appear to be trustworthy? What steps would you take to write regulations that make the agency appear to be credible to the regulated parties?

Policy Writer A: "I try to write so that I would understand exactly what is expected of me. Sometimes we are directed to write rules that are vague." [No further clarification was given.]

Policy Writer B: "Yes. We hold focus groups and workshops to ask providers what they want—intent. We held eight focus groups with field staff and providers and showed them the rule rough drafts."

Policy Writer C: "There is a lot of distrust among our providers. We have to be cognizant of distrust, but providers fail to understand that their goal should be to protect the children."

QUESTIONS ABOUT WRITING PROCESS

1. Who will review your draft regulation after you finish writing it?

Policy Writer A: [The policy writer then asked her administrative assistant to print a copy of the process chart, Cross-Agency Rulemaking Process Consolidation Project, and gave me a copy.]

Policy Writer B: "Other than the information on the flowchart that I gave you, CCL Rules Process, there is an internal review process within the CCL division. The rules are reviewed by the program director, legal, and routed to Child Protective Services for their comments, and finally routed to the Associate Commissioner for the Child Care Licensing Division. We had three workgroups to review the latest set of rules. We are considering holding other workgroups to update the stakeholders on the final document, which is about 300 pages. The number of rules increases as we translate and update them."

Policy Writer C: [The writer referred me to the Cross-Agency Rulemaking Process Consolidation Project chart.]

2. How would you describe your own personal writing process? For example, do you begin with research, use templates, or write collaboratively in a meeting setting?

Policy Writer A: "Most of my writing is collaborative writing and done face to face. I type up my notes in Microsoft Word after meetings where we discuss rule changes. Then I share notes with the rest of the group to make sure that I understood what was stated. Then I write rule drafts. I start with the answer, and then I write the question or title last. For the daycare rules, I worked in a large group to understand definitions such as 'facility,' 'permit holder,' and 'operation.' For example, in old regulations, we used terms such as 'registrant' and 'licensee,' but 'permit holder' is more inclusive. Other terms that needed clarifying were "regular" and "frequent" referring to inspections. We defined these terms to mean a specific number of days—30 days. The legal staff was very supportive in our writing process and we came to a clear understanding about which words needed to be defined. We decided that if a word has a different meaning in the dictionary than our use of the word, then it needs to be defined by us in the regulation."

Policy Writer B: " I start by thinking about our mission. Primarily we need to consider the children and their voice, the licensing representations [field inspectors], providers, and legislators. [Policy Writer B stated that she considers her audiences' responses in the following order of importance: legislators, children, licensing representatives, and then providers.] I have an idea about what I want to say, what is important. A rule that speaks to the subject [content]. What are the important elements that I want to cover? Then I group the elements into three questions. Plain English makes writers ask themselves what they really mean. I still use subsections in the Plain English rules, like Roman numerals, but I'm not as concerned with the words with my educated audience."

Policy Writer C: "I think about information that I've gotten in the field at various times. I think about issues other divisions such as CPS are dealing with. I think about the internal stakeholders."

3. Describe your work environment?

Policy Writer A: [I observed that Policy writer A has a cubicle, computer, table, window view, cabinets with books and resources] Policy Writer A uses MS Word to draft rules and Microsoft Excel to capture data on the public comments she receives. She received 16,000 comments on the daycare revisions and stored them in a spreadsheet by type of comment and rule number. [Policy Writer A is the only person with access to this spreadsheet, which is located on the hard disk of her desktop, and she is not sure agency staff would want the large document tying up the server space.]

Policy Writer B: [I observed that Policy Writer B has a cubicle with a table, computer, window, and cabinets with several reference books.] Policy Writer B conducts a lot of research on the Internet, consults with others, and has in-office references, specifically research that discusses standards and rationale like "Caring for Our Children," which comments on standards from other states. She showed me references that have implications for all children, like the Council on Accreditation Policies and Procedures, which recommends standards for residential childcare. She also looks at other states. "California has standards on water activities that we may need to borrow from."

Policy Writer C: [I observed that Policy Writer C had a cubicle with a computer, window, and file cabinets.] She states that she uses Microsoft Word, Excel, and Internet Explorer to conduct research about other state agencies. She states that e-mail is very important in collaborating with other policy writers. Policy Writer C showed me a derivation table. "We use derivation tables, which we create in Microsoft Excel, to keep track rule changes. These tables tell us where rules originate, why we create a rule, the difference between old and new rules and standards, and puts old and new language back to back. We can see how the rule has changed by looking at the table. Disposition tables tell us."

4. What is your experience with writing in Plain English or legalese? Which writing style do you prefer?

Policy Writer A: "I believe Plain English is more effective. Legalese requires more thought [by the audience]. There is consideration of a new 'Rationale' document that providers can use that includes the rationale or interpretation of the regulation. I've never written in legalese."

Policy Writer B: "Plain English is difficult to write. It's hard to try to write something that is clear and not too prescriptive. We don't want to box ourselves in and need flexibility to use judgment, but we feel much better about the final product with Plain English. Legalese has too much wiggle room, it's not clear, but it's easier to write. I wrote regulations in legalese before switching to Plain English. [Policy Writer B's provider audience's rules have to have enough flexibility to allow for different organizational structures of facilities.]

Policy Writer C: "Instead of making large-scale revisions to all rules at once, I'd like to rewrite rules over a four-to-five-year period so that they can compare the new and old style to see the benefits of Plain English. In previous positions in state agencies, attorneys wrote the regulations. I've never written in legalese. I think legalese can be too complicated for our providers and easier to interpret in several ways."

APPENDIX IV

The Focus Group Meeting

The facilitator read the following scenario and instructions.

> Facilitator:
> "Congratulations, you've just inherited a daycare center in the Austin area. One of your staff members informs you that your business is regulated by a state agency and that you must follow state regulations. Your staff person gives you a couple of regulations and informs you that daycares are inspected and that you must follow regulations to avoid being written up for non-compliances. Now, take 5 to 10 minutes to read the regulations (A and B) on the first page. Both of these regulations are about the same thing but written in different styles. Feel free to make notes on the handouts." [Note: The example regulations that I used in the focus group address similar topics, but are not word-for-word translations of the original regulations. In many instances, several Plain English regulations are needed to cover the content of one legalese regulation.]

The participants then read the following text from page 1 of the 2-page handout. Please read the following regulations:

> A.
> RULE §725.2038. Notification of Non-compliance. The facility is entitled to written notification of any non-compliance with the conditions of probation or evaluation, including non-compliance with standards and/or the law.
>
> **Source**: Texas Administrative Code: Title 40 Social Services and Assistance, Part 2. West Group, 2001.
>
> B.
> RULE §745.8601 What happens if I am deficient in a minimum standard, rule, law, specific term of my permit, or condition of evaluation, probation, or suspension?
> We may make recommendations and/or impose remedial actions for any deficiency.
>
> **Source**: Office of the Texas Secretary of State. Texas Administrative. Title 40 Social Services and Assistance, Part 19, Chapter 745, Subchapter K, Division 1. Section. 745.8601.

140 / FROM BLACK CODES TO RECODIFICATION

After all participants stated that they had read the regulations, the facilitator asked the following questions. The participants' responses are documented under each question.

Question 1: Which of these regulations is easier to understand? Why?

Subject A: "Rule B is easier to understand because it was expressed in everyday language, as if the person was speaking with us."

Subject F: "Rule A was because it is the opposite [of what of Subject A stated] because it does not speak directly to you, but it is in a standard format that is easier to understand."

Subject D: "Rule B because it is straightforward and says what would happen if it were to take place."

Subject B: "Rule A because I had to drop out some words that I thought were unnecessary to understand B."

Subject C: "Rule B because it is in laymans terms and plain language because you wouldn't have to guess about what a word means."

Question 2. Are there any words in either of these regulations that should be defined to make it easier for you and your new staff to follow?

[I asked Subject B which words he needed to "drop out" to understand Rule B.]

Subject B: "I dropped some words to understand the question part. The question part is too wordy."

Subject F: "Impose" would have to be changed."

Subject B: "The double negatives, like non-noncompliance. Rule A sounds like they're trying to make it difficult to understand. Both look like the writer is trying to make it more difficult to understand."

Question 3: What do you think of that fact that in the first regulation, you (the new owner) are referred to as a facility whereas in the second regulation, the regulation writer refers to you in first-person?

Subject D: "If you are the owner, then they're speaking in first-person to you. While if you, as the owner, have a manager to manage your facility, the nonquestion answer format without the "you" covers both bases; they could be addressing the owner or the facility by saying "you" are responsible for the facility. So if you use the words "I" or "you," the responsibility is placed on whoever reads it."

Subject B: "In most cases, rules are not read, because it seems very cold and it would cause a person not to read the rule, while the second [Rule B] seems more likely to encourage a person to read it or at least be aware of it. The first [Rule A] reminds me of the mentality in Communist Russia, where you must do this and that's it."

Subject F: "Rule A is trying to be more inclusive of different things, and government regulations are usually more punitive because regulations are written to make a person do things. I can't see a government entity limiting itself the way B does. It is possible to put both "I" and "facility" in the rule to cover the facility and the owner."

Subject D: "In the . . . rules, if I didn't follow them it would possibly put us out of business. Most rules are written to extract money from us. Rules are written with administrative penalties assigned to them."

Question 4: Does the fact that the writer is referring to you personally make you more trustful or willing to cooperate?

Subject F: "It makes me more trustful."

Subject B: "It would make me go back and read it."

Subject B: "Rule A starts out with a punitive tone, no questions, if, and, or buts about it. How is that a turn-on to start off negative? The tone in B opens up with a question that makes you feel better about the rule and even acknowledge that you may be deficient and that they are willing to work with you."

> Facilitator:
> Now, take 5 to10 minutes to read the regulations (D and C) on the second page. Both of these regulations are about the same thing, but written in different styles.

The participants then read the following text from the second page of the 2-page handout.
Please read the following regulations:

C.
RULE §745.8403 What is the purpose of an inspection?
The purpose of an inspection is to:
(1) Verify compliance with licensing statutes, rules, and minimum standards;
(2) Assess the risk to children in facilities;
(3) Evaluate whether the operation is subject to regulation;
(4) Assist the provider in identifying problems contributing to violations of licensing statutes, rules, and minimum standards;
(5) Offer technical assistance; and
(6) Gather information as part of an investigation.

Source: Office of the Texas Secretary of State. Title 40 Social Services and Assistance, Part 19, Chapter 745, Subchapter L, Division 1. Section. 745.8403.

D.
RULE §725.2001. Inspection Visits. Unregulated and regulated facility/ registered/ or listed home staff must admit licensing staff and not delay or obstruct licensing staff from making inspections during hours of operation.

(1) Although the licensee/registrant/listee of a regulated facility may choose to limit children to certain areas of the structure, the licensee/ registrant/listee must allow the licensing representative to inspect any area of the facility/registered or listed family home that affects or could affect the health, safety, or well-being of the children in care. When inspection is refused, obstructed, or delayed by facility/registered or listed family home staff to the extent that licensing staff cannot carry out their responsibility, the facility/registered or listed family home shall be advised that these actions are in violation of the Human Resources Code, §42.044(a), and that the license/certificate/registration/listing may be revoked and/or legal action requested if resistance continues.
(2) More than one inspection visit may be necessary to complete an investigation or make a determination of compliance with licensing rules and standards.

Source: Texas Administrative Code: Title 40 Social Services and Assistance, Part 2. West Group, 2001.

After all participants stated that they had read the regulations, the facilitator asked the following questions. The participants' responses are documented under each question.

Question 1: Which of these regulations is easier to understand? Why?

Subject C: "When I read D, I visualized a stuffed shirt person with a cattle prod. I can see myself dreading that person coming in. In C, I saw a person coming in wanting to help me succeed. D is difficult to read because it runs long."

Subject B: "The second regulation [Rule D] has to be broken down several times. The second regulation sounds like we're here to hurt you. The second one sounds like it's opening up as possibilities to be punitive and the regulator is not sure of what might happen. The second one sounds as if they'll figure out a way to hurt the business. The first one sounds as if it's a wide open situation, an assessment."

Subject F: "The second one [Rule D] favors the regulated agency."

Question 2: Are there any words in either of the regulations that should be defined to make it easier for you and your new staff to follow?

Subject B: "Words like 'unregulated/regulated' allows for ambiguity, and that in itself tends to leave open some kind of action. It tends to lean toward the agency. All of the slashes seem to make it seem like there is no end to it. As a layperson, I think it is poorly written. An attorney might say that it is a great rule."

Subject C: "'Unregulated' lets me know that if my business is unregulated that I shouldn't be in business. How can you function as an unregulated facility?"

Subject B: "Define obstruct. Anything that looks as if they don't want to define what is it makes it unclear."

Subject F: "Words are definable; it just depends on who defines it. This leaves the door wide open for interpretation."

Subject C: "The whole regulation D is written to oppose you. Why would an unregulated facility be mentioned?"

Subject D: "I operate both an unregulated and a regulated facility and you're better off to operate a regulated facility and let them in. In an . . . facility, you don't have to apply for a license, but someone in the community may report you thinking you're supposed to be regulated and they come out to inspect . . . to make sure that you're out of compliance even though you're not supposed to be regulated. They look at the number of . . . I'm licensed for in the regulated facility. So my licensed facility hinges on my unregulated facility. Are there regulations for regulated and unregulated?"

Note: Most of the group thinks the first rule makes more sense because it doesn't go into any discussion of an unregulated facility. There is confusion about what an "unregulated facility" is and why it is mentioned if unregulated facilities are exempt from regulation.

Subject C: "They have a way to get you no matter what, even if you don't let them in because you're unregulated. Wow!" [The group laughs.]

Subject B: "In daycare centers, it's my understanding that once you're licensed, you're unregistered or listed. There are still regulations for all types of daycare facilities."

Question 3: Is there language in either of the regulations that sounds like the regulation writer is trying to help the daycare owner?

Subject C: "All of the language in the first regulation seems helpful. It's my business and you laid it out for me so that I can keep my business in compliance."

Subject B: "The first regulation lists everything that needs to be listed: 'assist,' 'compliance,' 'offer assistance,' 'information.'"

Subject A: "The second regulation tells you what they are going to do with you and for you; it introduces their job title to you."

Subject F: "The first one is clear. C covers everything that D is saying and C seems helpful in nature."

Subject B: "The first one [Rule C] sounds like I'm going to do this for you. Two [Rule D] sounds like I'm going to do it *to* you as many times as possible."

Subject B: "Rule D leaves a lot of room for personalities to show their heads. 'And/or' and 'resistance' sound as if it is your mother pointing her finger at you. Resistance is futile, and I'm coming at you. The first line, they refer to 'refusal' before anyone even said they would refuse it." [The group laughs.]

Subject D: "I get C and D. They e-mail rules in a question-and-answer format, and they mail the other type to the providers on the list. So there are times we when we get it in both formats; I prefer C."

Question 4: Do you believe that regulation writers purposely write in a manner to confuse the business owner?

Subject B: "I believe that regulation writers purposely write to confuse business owners."

[Several others nod their heads in agreement.]

Subject B: "Many times regulations are written by attorneys to cover the organizations' responsibilities as opposed to being written in a manner that the layperson can better comply. If there are actions taken against the facility, the agency has their bases covered. I'm involved in six lawsuits, and the burden is always on the plaintiff to prove that there was something that allows for ambiguity. It is written in a way that closes the door to persons on the outside. These words lend themselves to ambiguity so that when you're in court they're covered; they place you in 'the exception of' category."

Question 5: Do you trust regulation writers to enforce these regulations equally on African American business owners?

[Five of the six participants shook their heads suggesting that they didn't, but Subject B articulated an opinion.]

Subject B: "Regulation writers know that a lot of blacks are starting off 10 feet behind. They can't care that in any business we're going to be playing catch up."

Subject F: "Government regulators or enforcers are motivated by how many fines they can place on you. They are bonused by how many fines they can place on you. I can imagine that daycare facilities and home health care facilities are bonused on how many they can get. The people who write these rules are trying to help the enforcers get these bonuses."

Subject B: "When I get a bunch of rules, I take them to a lawyer first."

Subject F: "Sounds like you need an attorney to interpret the regulations for you."

Subject B: "It is economics; we are at the lowest level of the economic ladder. We don't have the ability to get attorneys. We have the economic obstacle to everything we're trying to do. Is it not written so a layperson can help you comply, but it is written in a way that an attorney has to help you. The regulation writers know that there is going to be a shortfall. We are at the bottom, and everyone in this country knows it. It is just a matter that 'they' are unable to hide under the radar. The regulation writer knows that too often we don't have the ability to get the legal teams to help us once we fight, once we've violated the regulation."

Subject B: "Rule C gives the impression that we're going to provide some technical assistance. Every one of those words in D with a slash has a drop-down screen that seems like they link to some other catch. Rules are linked, and you have to have a battery of, not one, lawyers to defend yourself, and even they have problems. Attorneys still have problems; what chance do black people have to overcome legalese?"

[At this point, I asked if anyone disagreed? And everyone nodded their heads suggesting that they did agree with Subject B.]

Subject F: "We're all black aren't we?"

[No one voiced that they believed that African American business owners are not at a disadvantage.]

Question 6: Research shows that African Americans are less trusting of the government than other racial and ethnic groups. Do you believe that the way regulations are written may contribute to this trust or are there other factors?

Subject F: "I didn't know that they did that kind of research. Both, the way regulations are written does contribute to this fact. Are African Americans involved in writings regulations in the first place? Does anyone know of a black regulation writer?"

[No one responded.]

Subject B: "Not that African Americans don't understand the rules. We have to look at the history and how they've been changed and modified. Since slavery ended, we've learned how to play the rules, and they overlook the rules, don't play by them, or change them. They will boldface ignore what the rule says."

Subject D: "I try to look at it as being applied as equally across the board knowing that's not true. We were able to get enough facility owners to get the state to get a standard where all of the inspectors are trained to look at the same things when they came out and we were effective in getting that done. They would come in my place and look at certain things and go somewhere else look at other things. Now they use a checklist. The enforcement of rule is misapplied."

Subject F: "It is the way the rule is written that gives them the leeway to misapply the regulation."

Subject B: "Then we have to go back and show how it was misapplied. We're fighting the same battle we've been fighting for a hundred years, and most of the time it's overapplied on us."

    Facilitator:
    "Well, that's about all we have time for this morning. Thanks again for participating in this study."

References

Aberbach, J. D., & Walker, J. L. (1970). Political trust and racial ideology. *American Political Science Review, 64*, 1199–1219.

Abney, F. G., & Hutcheson, J. D., Jr. (1981). Race, representation, trust: Changes in attitudes after the election of a black mayor. *Public Opinion Quarterly, 45,* 91–101.

Acosta, T. (2001, June 6). Juneteenth. *The handbook of Texas online.* The Texas State Historical Association. Retrieved 12/09/07.
http://tshaonline.org/handbook/online/articles/JJ/lkj1.html

Alkebulan, A. A. (2003). The spiritual essence of African American rhetoric. In R. L. Jackson, II & E. B. Richardson (Eds.), *Understanding African American rhetoric: Classical origins to contemporary innovations.* New York: Routledge.

Alford, K. (2003, September 30). African American History Lecture, Texas Tech University, Lubbock.

Aristotle. (1991). *On rhetoric.* (G. A. Kennedy, Trans.). New York: Oxford University Press.

Baake, K. (2003). *Metaphors and knowledge: The challenges of writing science.* Albany, NY: SUNY Press.

Bacon, F. (1858). *The works of Francis Bacon* (Vol. V). J. Spedding, R. Ellis, & D. Health (Eds.). London: Longman and Co.

Banks, A. (2006). *Race, rhetoric, and technology: Searching for higher ground.* Mahwah, NJ: Lawrence Erlbaum Associates.

Barker, T. (1998). *Writing software documentation: A task oriented approach.* Needham Heights, MA: Allyn & Bacon.

Barr, A. (1996). *Black Texans: A history of African Americans in Texas, 1528–1995* (2nd ed.). Norman, OK: University of Oklahoma Press.

Bernstein, D. E. (2001). *Only one place to redress: African Americans, labor regulations, and the courts from reconstruction to the new deal.* Durham, NC: Duke University Press.

Bizzell, P., & Herzberg B. (Eds.). (2001). Rhetorica ad herennium. *The rhetorical tradition: Readings from classical times to the present.* Boston/New York: Bedford/St. Martins.

Black, H. C. (1990). *Black's law dictionary with pronunciations* (6th ed.). St. Paul, MN: West Publishing Company.

Bothamely, J. (2002). *Dictionary of theories.* New York: Visible Ink Press.

Bureau of Labor Statistics. (1923, September). *Laws of Texas relating to labor.* Austin, TX.
Bureau of Labor Statistics. (1947, September). *Laws of Texas relating to labor.* Austin, TX.
Bureau of National Affairs. (1964). *State fair employment laws and their administration: Texts, federal-state cooperation, prohibited acts.* Washington, DC: BNA.
Bush, G. W. (2005, September 15). Transcript of speech in Jackson Square, New Orleans, LA. Retrieved 12/09/07. http://www.cnn.com/2005/POLITICS/09/15/bush.transcript/
Butler, J. P. (1867). Report to Lieutenant L. P. Richardson, January 31, 1867. In M. F. Williams (Ed.), *Records of the assistant commissioner for the state of Texas, bureau of refugees, freedmen, and abandoned lands, letters sent, 1865–1869* (Vol. 1, pp. 1–8, pp. 1–12, RG 105, microfilm publication M821, reel 24).
CBS/Associated Press. (2006, June 1). *Katrina report blames levees: Army corps of engineers: "We've had a catastrophic failure."* Retrieved 12/09/07. http://www.cbsnews.com/stories/2006/06/01/national/main1675244.shtml
CNN.com. (2006). *Fortune 500 2006: Our annual ranking of America's largest corporations.* Retrieved 12/09/07. http://money.cnn.com/magazines/fortune/fortune500/full_list/
Cicero, M. T. (1988). *De oratore.* (E. W. Sutton, Trans.). Cambridge, MA: Harvard University Press.
Cicero, M. T. (1998). *The laws.* (N. Rudd, Trans.). New York: Oxford University Press.
Cooter, R., & Ulen, T. (1988). *Law and economics.* Glenview, IL: Scott, Foresman, and Company.
Crouch, B. A. (1999). To enslave the rising generation: The Freedmen's Bureau and the Texas black code. In P. A. Cimbala & R. M. Miller (Eds.), *The Freedmen's Bureau and reconstruction.* New York: Fordham.
Derrida, J. (1982). *Margins in philosophy.* (A. Bass, Trans.). Chicago: University of Chicago Press.
Dombrowski, P. M. (2000). Survey of ethics in communication and rhetoric. *Ethics in Technical Communication.* Needham Heights, MA: Allyn & Bacon.
Dorman, J. (1988). Shaping the popular image of post-reconstruction American blacks: The "Coon Song" phenomenon of the gilded age. *American Quarterly, 40,* 450–471.
DuBois, W. E. B. (1901). The Freedman's Bureau. *Atlantic Monthly, 97,* 354–365.
DuBois, W. E. B. (2003). *The souls of black folk.* New York: Modern Library Edition.
Ede, L., & Lunsford, A. (1997). Audience addressed/audience invoked: The role of audience in composition theory and pedagogy. In V. Villanueva, Jr. (Ed.), *Cross-talk in comp theory: A reader* (pp. 77–95). Urbana, IL: National Council of Teachers of English.
11th Texas Legislature. (1866a). *Chapter CXXVIII. An act to define and declare the rights of persons lately known as slaves, and free persons of color. 1861–1866, 5, 1049–1050, 1866.* Denton, TX: University of North Texas Libraries. Retrieved May 29, 2005, from Gammel's Laws of Texas http://texinfo.library.unt.edu/lawsoftexas/contents.html
11th Texas Legislature. (1866b). *Chapter CXI. An act to define the offence of vagrancy, and to provide for the punishment of vagrants. 1861-1866, 5, 1020-1022, 1866.* Denton, TX: University of North Texas Libraries. Retrieved May 29, 2005, from Gammel's Laws of Texas http://texinfo.library.unt.edu/lawsoftexas/contents.html
11th Texas Legislature. (1866c). *Chapter LXXXII. An act to provide for the punishment of persons tampering with, persuading or enticing away, harboring, feeding or secreting*

laborers or apprentices, or for employing laborers or apprentices under contract of service to other persons. 1861–1866, 5, 998–999, 1866. Denton, TX: University of North Texas Libraries. Retrieved May 29, 2005, from http://texinfo.library.unt.edu/lawso Gammel's Laws of Texas ftexas/contents.html

11th Texas Legislature. (1866d). *Chapter LXXX. An act regulating contracts for labor, 1861-1866, 5, p. 994–997, 1866.* Denton, TX: University of North Texas Libraries. Retrieved May 29, 2005, from Gammel's Laws of Texas http://texinfo.library.unt.edu/lawsoftexas/contents.html

11th Texas Legislature. (1866e). *Chapter LXXIII. An act to amend an act to adopt and establish a penal code for the state of Texas, approved August 28, 1856, and to repeal certain portions thereof, 1861-1866, 5, 988–989, 1866.* Denton, TX: University of North Texas Libraries. Retrieved May 29, 2005, from Gammel's Laws of Texas http://texinfo.library.unt.edu/lawsoftexas/contents.html

11th Texas Legislature. (1866f). *Chapter LXIII. An act establishing a general apprentice law, and defining the obligations of master and mistress and apprentice, 1861-1866, 5, 979-981, 1866.* Denton, TX: University of North Texas Libraries. Retrieved May 29, 2005, from Gammel's Laws of Texas http://texinfo.library.unt.edu/lawsoftexas/contents.html

Elling, R. (1997, October). Revising safety instructions with focus groups. *Journal of Business and Technical Communication, 11*(4), 451–468.

Elliot, E. (1989). The veil, the mask, and the invisible empire: Representations of race in the gilded age. *Rivista Di Studi Anglo-Americani, 5,* 11–27.

Foucault, M. (1972). *The archaeology of knowledge and the discourse on language.* (A. M. S. Smith, Trans.). New York: Pantheon Books.

Frooman, H. (1981). Lawyers and readability. *Journal of Business Communication, 18,* 45–51.

Glover, T. (1992). Trust, distrust, and feminist theory. *Hypatia, 7,* 16–33.

Gore, A. (1998, August 5). Remarks by Vice President Al Gore as Prepared Second Plain English Award. National partnership for reinventing government. Retrieved 12/09/07, from http://govinfo.library.unt.edu/npr/library/speeches/080598.html

Gregory, E. M. (2002a). Letter to Major General O. O. Howard, 18 Apr 1866. In H. Ide (Ed.), *Records of the assistant commissioner for the state of Texas, Bureau of Refugees, Freedmen, and Abandoned Lands, 1865–1869, letters sent* (Vol. 1, pp. 192–195). National Archives, RG 105, microfilm M821, reel 1. http://freepages.military.rootsweb.com/~pa91/ftxls00.html

Gregory, E. M. (2002b). Letter to Major General O. O. Howard, 31 January 1866. In H. Ide (Ed.), *Records of the assistant commissioner for the state of Texas, Bureau of Refugees, Freedmen, and Abandoned Lands, 1865–1869, letters sent* (Vol. 1, pp. 122–125). National Archives, RG 105, microfilm M821, reel 1. http://freepages.military.rootsweb.com/~pa91/ftxls00.html

Gregory, E. M. (2002c). Letter to Benjamin Harris, 20 January 1866. In H. Ide (Ed.), *Records of the assistant commissioner for the state of Texas, Bureau of Refugees, Freedmen, and Abandoned Lands, 1865–1869, letters sent* (Vol. 1, pp. 109–113). National Archives, RG 105, microfilm M821, reel 1. http://freepages.military.rootsweb.com/~pa91/ftxls00.html

Gregory, E. M. (2002d). Report, 9 December, 1865. In H. Ide (Ed.), *Records of the assistant commissioner for the state of Texas, Bureau of Refugees, Freedmen, and Abandoned Lands, 1865–1869, letters sent* (Vol. 1, pp. 65–70). National Archives,

RG 105, microfilm M821, reel 1.
http://freepages.military.rootsweb.com/~pa91/ftxls00.html
Gregory, E. M. (2002e). Circular letter, 17 October 1865. In H. Ide (Ed.), *Records of the assistant commissioner for the state of Texas, Bureau of Refugees, Freedmen, and Abandoned Lands, 1865-1869, letters sent* (Vol. 1, pp. 20–21). National Archives, RG 105, microfilm M821, reel 1.
http://freepages.military.rootsweb.com/~pa91/ftxls00.html
Gregory, E. M. (2002f). Letter to Benjamin Harris, 21 September 1865. In H. Ide (Ed.), *Records of the assistant commissioner for the state of Texas, Bureau of Refugees, Freedmen, and Abandoned Lands, 1865–1869, letters sent* (Vol. 1, pp. 109–113). National Archives, RG 105, microfilm M821, reel 1.
http://freepages.military.rootsweb.com/~pa91/ftxls00.html
Hague, B. N., & Loader B. (Eds.). (1999). *Digital democracy: Discourse and decision making in the information age.* London: Routledge.
Haynes, R. V. (2003, November 2). Houston Riot of 1917. *The handbook of Texas online.* The Texas State Historical Association. Retrieved 12/09/07.
http://tshaonline.org/handbook/online/articles//HH/jch4.html
Holtzblatt, K., & Beyer, H. (1996). *Contextual design: Principles and practice, in field methods casebook for software design.* D. Wixon & J. Ramey (Eds.). New York: Wiley.
Howell, S. E., & Fagan, D. (1988). Race and trust in government: Testing the political reality model. *Public Opinion Quarterly, 52,* 343–350.
Huddleston, J. D. (2001, June 6). Miriam Amanda Wallace Ferguson. *The handbook of Texas online.* The Texas State Historical Association. Retrieved 12/09/07.
http://tshaonline.org/handbook/online/articles/FF/ffe6.html
Johnson, R. R. (1998). *User-centered technology: A rhetorical theory for computers and other mundane artifacts.* Albany, NY: SUNY Press.
Kennedy, G. A. (1994). *A new history of classical rhetoric.* Princeton, NJ: Princeton University Press.
Kerwin, C. (1994). *Rulemaking: How government agencies write law and make policy.* Washington, DC: Congressional Quarterly Inc.
Knopf, K. A. (1991). *A lexicon of economics.* New York: Academic Press.
Lanham, R. (2003). *Analyzing prose* (2nd ed.). New York: Charles Scribner's Sons.
Lather, P. (1996). Troubling clarity: The politics of accessible language. *Harvard Educational Review, 66,* 525–545.
LeFevre, K. B. (1987). *Invention as a social act.* Carbondale, IL: Southern Illinois University Press.
Leopold, T. (2005). *'Louisiana 1927' A song and a tragedy.* Retrieved 12/09/07.
http://www.cnn.com/2005/SHOWBIZ/08/31/eye.ent.louisiana/
Lewis, D. L. (1995). *W. E. B. Dubois: A reader.* New York: Henry Holt & Company.
Logan, R. W. (1954). *The Negro in American life and thought: The nadir, 1877–1901.* New York: Dial Press, Inc.
Longinus. (1952). On the sublime. In L. Cooper (Ed. and Trans.), *The art of the writer: Essays, excerpts, and translations* (pp. 219–223). Ithaca, NY: Cornell University Press.
Longo, B. (1998, Winter). An approach for applying cultural study theory to technical writing research. *Technical Communication Quarterly, 7*(1), 53–73.
Longo, B. (2000). *Spurious coin: A history of science, management, and technical writing.* Albany, NY: SUNY Press.

Lowenstein, R. B. (1981). Forward to the fundamentals. *English Journal, 70*(3), 88–89.
MacNealy, M. S. (1999). *Strategies for empirical research in writing.* Needham Heights, MA: Allyn & Bacon.
Markel, M. (2004). *Technical communication,* (7th ed.). Boston: Bedford/St. Martin's.
Markel, M. (2006). *Technical communication,* (8th ed.). Boston: Bedford/St. Martin's.
Moneyhon, C. H. (2003, November 2). Black codes. *The handbook of Texas online.* Retrieved 12/09/07. http://tshaonline.org/handbook/online/articles/BB/jsb1.html
Murray, D. (1997). Teach writing as a process not product. In V. Villanueva, Jr. (Ed.), *Cross-talk in comp theory: A reader* (pp. 3–6). Urbana, IL: National Council of Teachers of English.
National Public Radio. (2000). *Americans distrust government, but want it to do more: Npr/Kaiser/Kennedy school poll point to paradox.* Retrieved 12/09/07. http://npr.org/programs/specials/poll/govt/summary.html
Obama, B. H. (2009). Memorandum, 21 January 2009. Transparency and open government. In *Federal Register, 74*(15), 4685-4686.
Office of the Texas Secretary of State. (2005a, May 1). Title 40 social services and assistance, Part 19, Chapter 745, Subchapter K, Division 1. Section. 745.8601. *Texas Administrative Code.* Retrieved 1/22/05.
http://www.sos.state.tx.us/tac/index.shtml
Office of the Texas Secretary of State. (2005b, May 1). Title 40 social services and assistance, Part 19, Chapter 745, Subchapter L, Division 1. Section. 745.8403. *Texas Administrative Code.* Retrieved 1/22/05.
http://www.sos.state.tx.us/tac/index.shtml
Okun, A. M. (1975). *Equality and efficiency: The big trade-off.* Washington, DC: The Brookings Institution.
Plainlanguage.gov. (2005, May 1). *Plain language: Improving communications from the federal government to the public.* Retrieved 12/09/07.
http://www.plainlanguage.gov/usingPL/government/index.php
Plato. (1970). *The laws.* (T. J. Saunders, Trans.). New York: Penguin Books.
Randolph, A. P. (1936, January). The trade union movement and the negro. *Journal of Negro Education, 5*(1) 54–58.
Rickard, T. A. (1920, 1923). *Technical writing* (2nd ed.). New York: John Wiley & Sons.
Rose, R. (1993). *Lesson-drawing in public policy: A guide to learning across time and space.* Chatham NJ: Chatham House.
Ross, S. M. (1994, Summer). A feminist perspective on technical communication action: Exploring how alternative worldviews affect environmental remediation efforts. *Technical Communication Quarterly, 3*(3), 325–342.
Royster, J. J. (Ed.). (1997). *Southern horrors and other writings: The anti-lynching campaign of Ida B. Wells, 1892–1900.* Boston: Bedford/St. Martin's.
Rude, C. D. (2004). Toward an expanded concept of rhetorical delivery: The uses of reports in public policy debates. *Technical Communication Quarterly, 13*(3), 271–288.
Securities and Exchange Commission. (1998). A plain English handbook: How to create clear SEC disclosure documents. Retrieved 12/09/07.
http://www.sec.gov/pdf/handbook.pdf
Shulman, S. W., Scholosberg, D., Zavestoski. S., & Courard-Hauri, D. (2003, Summer). Electronic rulemaking: A public participation research agenda for the social sciences. *Social Science Computer Review, 21*(2), 162.

Simmons, D. E., & Simmons, D. A. (1906). *Texas laws made plain: Laws and legal forms prepared for the use of farmers mechanics and business men.* Kansas City, MO: Bankers Law Publishers Company.

Simmons, D. E., & Simmons, D. A. (1921). *Texas laws made plain: Laws and legal forms prepared for the use of farmers mechanics and business men.* Kansas City, MO: Bankers Law Publishers Company.

Suleiman, L. P. (2003). Beyond cultural competence: Language access and Latino civil rights. *Child Welfare, 82*(2), 185–200.

Sullivan, D. (1994). Political-ethical implications of defining technical communication as practice. In P. Dombrowski (Ed.), *Humanistic aspects of technical communication.* Amityville, NY: Baywood.

Taylor, Q. (1998). *In search of the racial frontier: African American west, 1528–1990* New York: W. W. Norton.

Texas Administrative Code. (2001). *Title 40 social services and assistance,* Part 2. West Group.

Texas cops suspended for joking about club fire. (2005, March 7). *The Chicago Sun-Times.*

Thomas, V. M. (2000). *Freedom's children: The passage from emancipation to the great migration.* New York: Crown Publishers.

Thralls, C., & Blyler, N. R. (1993). The social perspective and pedagogy in technical communication. *Technical Communication Quarterly, 2*(3), 249–270.

Thrush, E. (1997). Multicultural issues in technical communication. In K. Staples & C. M. Ornatowski (Eds.), *Foundations for teaching technical communication theory, practice, and program design.* Greenwich, CT: Ablex Publishing Corporation.

Ting-Toomey, S. (1999). *Communicating across cultures.* New York: The Guilford Press.

12th Legislature of the State of Texas. (1871). *General laws of the twelfth legislature of the state of Texas. First session–1871.* Austin, TX.

United States Department of Commerce—Minority Business Development Agency. (2006, April 18). *African American owned businesses total 1.2 million and generate 89 million in revenues.* U.S. Department of Commerce News.

University of Chicago Law Review. (1970, Winter). *Title VII of the Civil Rights Acts of 1964 and minority group entry into the building trade unions.* Vol. 27, No. 2, pp. 328–358.

Walzer, A, E., & Gross, A. (1994, April). Positivists, postmodernists, Aristotelians, and the Challenger disaster. *College English, 56*(4), 420–433.

Washington, B. T. (1901). *Up from slavery.* New York: Penguin Books.

Wesley, C. H. (1939, Summer). Organized labor and the negro. *Journal of Negro Education, 8*(3), 449–461. The Present and Future Position of the Negro in the American Social Order.

West, C. (2004). *Democracy matters: Winning the fight against imperialism.* New York: Penguin Press.

Williams, J. (1986). Plain English: The remaining problems. *Visible Language, 20,* 166–173.

Index

Aberbach, Joel D., 16-17
Abney, F. Glen, 17-18
African Americans and veiled language/historical regulations, 1-3, 7-8, 13
  See also Black business owners, contemporary; Invention heuristic for regulatory writing; Texas *listings*
Ambiguous and abstract terms, 73-74, 87
Analyzing Prose (Lanham), 12
"An Approach for Applying Cultural Study Theory to Technical Writing Research" (Longo), 10
Apprenticeships, 42-44, 88, 98-102, 118-121, 126-127
Aristotle, 4, 5-6
Atlanta (GA), trust of government in, 18
"Audience Addressed/Audience Invoked: The Role of Audience in Composition Theory and Pedagogy" (Ede & Lunsford), 58
Austin (TX). *See* Black business owners, contemporary

Baier, Annette, 21
Baker, Houston, 1
Banks, Adam, 90
Barker, Thomas, 53
Barr, Alwyn, 45
Barrett, Gary, 121
Berlin, James, 83
Bias, researcher, 12
Bizzell, Patricia, 83

Black business owners, contemporary
  ambiguous terms, 73-74
  cooperative/uncooperative language, 77
  discriminatory language, 75-76
  Dot's Restaurant, 67
  facilitator (professional counselor), use of a, 69, 70
  flexibility in style and language, 77-78
  growth in number of, 68
  image of government personnel, 72
  Midtown Live, 67-68
  outsider participant not governed by texts under scrutiny, 70
  overview, 10
  participants in focus group study, 68-69
  police officers' lack of sympathy/sensitivity, 67-68
  public participation in regulation/policy development, 76, 79, 84
  punitive language, 76-77
  regulations under scrutiny by focus group, 70-71
  "Revising Safety Instructions with Focus Groups," 69
  trust in enforcement practices, lack of, 76
  wordiness in written contracts, 72-73
Black Registry, 68
Bloom's Taxonomy, 12
Blyler, Nancy, 10, 83
Bryant, Anthony M., 116
Burke, Karen, 55-56

Bush, George W., 19, 64
Butler, James, 23, 24-25, 32, 117-119

Capital City African-American Chamber of Commerce Newsletter, 68-69
CCL. *See* Child Care Licensing Division of the Texas Department of Family and Protective Services
Census, U.S., 68
Center for Political Studies, 18
Child Care Licensing Division of the Texas Department of Family and Protective Services, 7
   See also Texas agencies: challenge of evoking trust
Cicero, 3-5
Clarity and classical rhetoricians, 5
Classical rhetoricians and regulatory writing, 3-6
Clinton, Bill, 6
Coleman, Thereisa, 69
Collaborative nature of regulatory writing, 64, 132
Communicating Across Cultures (Ting-Toomey), 10-11
Consistency, reducing redundancy and increasing, 61, 87-88
Contextual inquiry
   audience, questions about, 132-134
   author, who is the, 130-131
   collaboration with other organizations and resources, 132
   defining terms, 49
   focus group study tied to, 11
   how do you write regulations?, 129-130
   revision process, describing the, 131
   trust, questions about, 134
   why do you write regulations?, 129
   writing process, questions about, 134-137
   See also Texas agencies: challenge of evoking trust
Contractual theory, 21
   See also Labor, contract-based
Cooperative/uncooperative language, 77

Cotton, laws concerning proper procedure for bailing, 40-42, 87
Crisis, The, 15
Crouch, Barry, 2, 16, 23, 24, 27, 35, 47, 115-118, 120, 121, 126
Cultural competence, 59-61, 80-82
Cultural-studies approach, 10-11, 23

Demetrius, 4
Derrida, Jacques, 113
Detroit (MI), trust of government in, 17
Difference principle, 21
Digital record of internal/external documentation of discussions that affect audiences, 86-87
Discourse analysis of Texas Black Codes of 1866, 12
   See also Texas Black Codes of 1866
Discriminatory regulations, 75-76
   See also Texas Black Codes of 1866
Dombrowski, Paul, 8
Dot's Restaurant, 67
Drafting/editing rules and subject-matter experts, 53-57, 61
DuBois, W. E. B., 1, 15, 24

Economic efficiency and equality, tradeoffs between, 21, 80
Ede, Lisa, 58, 60-61
Editing/drafting rules and subject-matter experts, 53-57, 61
Education and recently freed slaves, 117-118
Efficiency and equality, tradeoffs between, 21, 80
Electronic rulemaking (e-rulemaking), 90
Elling, Rien, 69
Elliot, Emory, 1-2
Employment laws/regulations for blacks/minorities, 46-47
   See also Labor, contract-based
Equality and economic efficiency, tradeoffs between, 21, 80

Equality and Efficiency: The Big Tradeoff (Okun), 21
Facilitator (professional counselor), use of a, 69, 70
Fagan, Deborah, 18-19
Federal Emergency Management Agency (FEMA), 19-20
Federal Register, 61
Feedback and rule writing, 61
Feminist theorists' interpretation of trust, 20-21
Ferguson, James, 64
Ferguson, Miriam, 64-65
Flexibility in style and language, 77-78, 86, 88-89
Focus group study, 11, 139-147
    See also Black business owners, contemporary
Foucault, Michel, 22, 83, 113
Freedmen's Bureau, Federal Government's, 23-24, 123, 125-126
Freedmen's Bureau, Texas, 116
    See also Texas Black Codes of 1866
Freire, Paulo, 83
Friedman, Milton, 21
Frooman, Hilary, 62

Glover, Trudy, 20-21, 76
Goals of regulations, 3, 5-6
Good faith/respect and studying the language of regulations, 17
Gore, Al, 6
Granger, Gordon, 112
Gregory, Edgar M., 15, 23, 24-25, 112, 117, 122-126

Habermas, Jurgen, 83
Harris, Benjamin G., 15, 124
Historical data, writers must maintain and reference, 86
"Houston" (DuBois), 15
Howard, O. O., 112, 117, 123
Howell, Susan E., 18-19
Hurricane Katrina, 19-20
Hutcheson, John D, Jr., 17-18

Identify the intended audience, 87
Implementation as a goal of regulation, 3, 5, 6
Interpretation as a goal of regulation, 3, 5-6
Invention heuristic for regulatory writing
    ambiguous and abstract terms, reduce, 87
    consistent language, use of, 87-88
    cultural factors considered in regulatory writing, 80-82
    digital record of internal/external documentation of discussions that affect audiences, 86-87
    distrustful audiences, identify and document concerns of, 86
    electronic rulemaking (e-rulemaking), 90
    equality and economic efficiency, tradeoffs between, 80
    flexibility in style and language, 86, 88-89
    future of regulatory writing, 89-91
    historical data, writers must maintain and reference, 86
    identify the intended audience, 87
    information new policy writers need to know, 82-83
    modifiers, avoid vague, 88
    nonessential clauses, don't hide important information in, 87
    overview, 10, 11-12
    prepositional phrases, avoid repetitive, 87
    public participation in regulation/policy development, 79, 90-91
    punitive language, 88
    referenced laws/statutes, identify, 88
    slash marks, avoid excessive use of, 87
    specific and broad, acknowledge writer's need to make a tradeoff between, 86
    style that meets needs of the government agency and the public, 83-85
    subject position you assign your audience, consider the, 88

[Invention heuristic for regulatory writing ambiguous and abstract terms, reduce] titles of the government staff inspecting regulated entity, identify the job, 87

Johnson, Lyndon B., 64
Johnson, Robert, 11
Journal of Negro Education, 45-46
Juneteenth (June 19), 112-113

Kaiser Family Foundation, 47
Kennedy School, 47
Kerwin, Cornelius M., 3

Labor, contract-based, 11, 42-47, 103-110, 121-127
See also Black business owners, contemporary
Lanham, Richard, 12, 13
Latinos with limited English proficiency, 59
Laws, The (Cicero), 4
Laws, The (Plato), 3, 120
Lee, Arthur, 36-37
LeFevre, Karen B., 22, 55-56
Legalese style of writing, 3, 62-65
See also Black business owners, contemporary; Texas *listings*
Lesson-Drawing in Public Policy (Rose), 56
Limited English proficiency (LEP) population, 59-60
Logan, Rayford, 35
Longinus, 13, 72
Longo, Bernadette, 10
Lunsford, Andrea, 58, 60-61
Lynchings, pamphlets published on, 35-36

Markel, Mike, 80
Melville, Herman, 1-2
Microsoft Excel, 56, 57
Microsoft Word, 55

Midtown Live, 67-68
Miller, Carolyn, 83
Minority Business Development Agency (MBDA), 68
Modifiers, avoid vague, 88
"Multicultural Issues in Technical Communication," 11-12
Murray, Donald, 55

Nagin, Ray, 20
National Black Chamber of Commerce, 68
National Public Radio/Kaiser Family Foundation/Kennedy School study/poll, 47
New Orleans (LA), trust of government in, 18-20
Nixon, Richard, 18
Nonessential clauses, don't hide important information in, 87
Notifying parties about proposed rule changes, 57, 61

Obama, Barack, 89
Okun, Arthur M., 21
On Rhetoric (Aristotle), 4
On Style (Demetrius), 4
On the Sublime (Longinus), 72
Orator, The (Cicero), 3

Plain English Handbook, A: How to Create SEC Documents, 61, 74
Plain English style of writing, 3, 6-9, 62-65
See also Invention heuristic for regulatory writing; Texas *listings; individual subject headings*
Plato, 3, 5, 120
Poetry and veiled language, 12-13
Police officers' lack of sympathy/sensitivity, 67-68
Political identity, African Americans having a strong group, 19-20, 75-76

"Political Trust and Racial Ideology"
(Aberbach & Walker), 17
"Positivists, Postmodernists, Aristotelians and the Challenger Disaster" (Walzer & Gross), 5
Prepositional phrases, avoid repetitive, 87
Prescribing as a goal of regulation, 3, 5, 6
"Present and Future Position of the Negro in the American Social Order, The" (Wesley), 46
Prewriting, 55
Public participation in regulation/policy development, 18, 22, 58-59, 76, 79, 84, 90-91
  See also Black business owners, contemporary
Punitive language, 76-77, 88

"Race, Representation, and Trust: Changes in Attitudes After the Election of a Black Mayor" (Hutcheson & Abney), 18, 76
Race and veiled language in historical regulations, 1-3, 7-8, 13
  See also Black business owners, contemporary; Invention heuristic for regulatory writing; Texas *listings*
"Racial Differences in Political Conceptualization" (Hagner & Pierce), 19
Randolph, A. Philip, 45-46
Rawls, John, 21
Record (digital) of internal/external documentation of discussions that affect audiences, 86-87
Redundancy, increasing consistency and reducing, 61, 87-88
Referenced laws/statutes, identify, 88
Respect/good faith and studying the language of regulations, 17
"Revising Safety Instructions with Focus Groups" (Elling), 69
Rhetorica ad Herennium Book IV, 4-6
Richards, Ann, 64
Richardson, J. P., 117, 119
Rickard, T. A., 41

Ross, Susan M., 83
Rude, Carolyn, 13
Rulemaking: How Government Agencies Write Law and Make Policy (Kerwin), 3

Sharecropping, 35-37
Simmons, D. A., 41, 42
Simmons, D. E., 37, 39, 41, 42
Slash marks, avoid excessive use of, 87
Slave Narratives of Texas, The, 112
Social action, the relationship of text to, 13
Souls of Black Folk (DuBois), 1, 75-76
State Fair Employment Laws and their Administration: Operations Manual Complementing the Civil Rights Act of 1964, 46
Strock, Lt. Gen. Carl, 20
Subject position you assign your audience, consider the, 88
Suleiman, Layla P., 59, 60
Sullivan, Dale, 49
"Survey of Ethics in Communication and Rhetoric," 8

Tacit knowledge, 57
  See also Texas laws and tacit laws
Taylor, Quintard, 35
Technical Communication (Markel), 80
Technical Writing, 41
Texas agencies: challenge of evoking trust
  artifacts collected during contextual inquiry study, 52
  Child Care Licensing Division of the Texas Department of Family and Protective Services, 50-51
  children, best interests of the, 60
  collaborative nature of regulatory writing, 64
  consistency, reducing redundancy and increasing, 61
  cultural competence, 59-61
  defining what a rule is, 55

[Texas agencies: challenge of evoking trust]
  drafting/editing rules and subject-matter experts, 53-57, 61
  external stakeholders involvement, 58-59
  feedback and rule writing, 61
  flowchart, CCL Rule Process, 53, 54
  internal stakeholders involvement, 58
  notifying parties about proposed rule changes, 57, 61
  overview, 9-10
  overview of contextual inquiry process, 51
  Plain English *vs.* legalese style of writing, 62-65
  process meeting with group of policy writers, 52-53
  tacit knowledge, 57
  writing tasks, analysis of regulatory, 53-65
Texas Black Codes of 1866
  African Americans and contract-based labor as focus of, 11
  apprentice law, 98-102, 118-121, 126-127
  Butler, James, 23
  codes that were analyzed, 22-23
  discourse analysis of, 12, 24, 25, 127
  distrust, examples in Codes that evoke, 27-29, 32
  education and recently freed slaves, 117-118
  freedmen representing the audience who could read/protect their own rights, 81
  Freedmen's Bureau, Federal Government's, 23-24
  intergovernmental conflicts lead to blacks' confusion, 15-16, 24-25
  labor, contract-based, 103-110, 121-127
  language that evokes trust/distrust, identifying, 25-27
  nondiscriminatory facade, 47
  overview, 9
  Plain English *vs.* legalese, 93-127

[Texas Black Codes of 1866]
  primary and secondary audiences for, 23
  race and race relations in Texas, 2-3, 93-95, 112-114
  repealing of the, 35
  rhetorical analysis of Plain English and legalese, 111-127
  "To Enslave the Rising Generation: The Freedman's Bureau and the Texas Black Code," 23
  trust, examples in Codes that evoke, 30-33
  vagrancy laws, 95-98, 114-118
Texas laws and tacit laws
  apprenticeship and contract labor, redefining, 42-44
  overview, 9
  sharecropping, 35-37
  State Fair Employment Laws and their Administration: Operations Manual Complementing the Civil Rights Act of 1964, 46
  Texas Laws Made Plain: Laws and Forms Prepared for Farmers Mechanics and Business Men, 37-44
  Texas Laws Relating to Labor of 1923, 40-42
  trust in government, rationale for a contemporary study of black, 46-47
  union laws and practices, 45-46
  voting, 44-45
  Wells, Ida B., 35-36
Texas Laws Made Plain: Laws and Forms Prepared for Farmers Mechanics and Business Men, 37-44, 87, 88
Texas Laws Relating to Labor of 1923, 40-42
Texas legislature (76th in 1999) and regulatory review, 7
Texas Register, 50, 52, 61
Texas Register Format and Style Guide, 61
Thralls, Charlotte, 10, 83
Thrush, Emily, 12
Ting-Toomey, Stella, 10, 24, 61, 72
Titles of the government staff inspecting regulated entity, identify the job, 87

"To Enslave the Rising Generation: The Freedmen's Bureau and the Texas Black Code" (Crouch), 23, 121
Traditional styles of regulatory writing, 3-6
Trust, identifying discourse markers of, 17-22, 76, 134
  See also Invention heuristic for regulatory writing; Texas agencies: challenge of evoking trust; Texas Black Codes of 1866
Twain, Mark, 1

Unions and tacit laws in Texas, 45-46
User-centered methodology, 11

Vagrancy laws, 95-98, 114-118
"Veil, the Mask, and the Invisible Empire, The: Representations of Race in Gilded Age" (Elliot), 1
Veiled language in historical regulations, race and, 1-3, 7-8, 13
  See also Black business owners, contemporary; Invention heuristic for regulatory writing; Texas *listings*
Villager, 68
Voting and tacit laws in Texas, 44-45

Walker, Jack L., 16-17
Wallace, Webster, 36
Washington, Booker T., 17
Wells, Ida B., 35-36
Wesley, Charles H., 46
West, Cornell, 1, 2
Williams, Joseph, 50
Williams, Nora L., 37
Wordiness in written contracts, 72-73
Writing process and contextual inquiry, 134-137